The BalleCore® Workout

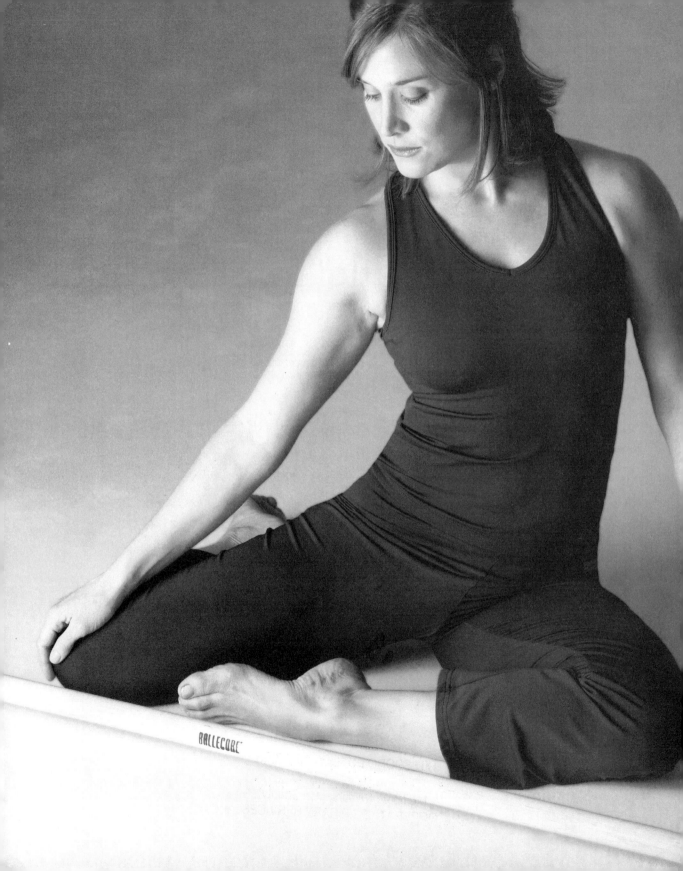

THE BALLECORE®

WORKOUT

Integrating Pilates, Hatha Yoga, and Ballet in an Innovative Exercise Routine for All Fitness Levels

Molly Weeks

BALLANTINE BOOKS • NEW YORK

Author's Note: This book proposes a program of exercise recommendations for the reader to follow. However, you should consult a qualified medical professional (and, if you are pregnant, your ob/gyn) before starting this or any other fitness program. As with any diet or exercise program, if you experience any discomfort, stop immediately and consult your physician.

A Ballantine Book
Published by The Random House Publishing Group

Copyright © 2005 by BalleCore, LIC

www.ballantinebooks.com

LIBRARY OF CONGRESS CATALOGING-IN-PUBLICATION DATA
Weeks, Molly
  The BalleCore workout: integrating Pilates, hatha yoga, and ballet in innovative
exercise for all fitness levels / Molly Weeks.—1st ed.
    p. cm.
  Includes index.
  ISBN 0-345-47190-3 *3227 8094 8/05*
    1. Exercise. 2. Physical fitness. 3. Pilates method. 4. Hatha yoga. 5. Ballet. I. Title.

RA 781.W374 2005
613. 7'1—dc22

                                                                    2004048852

Designed by BTDNYC

Photographs by Angela Sterling

Manufactured in the United States of America

First Edition

10 9 8 7 6 5 4 3 2 1

ACKNOWLEDGMENTS

I would like to thank the following people who have assisted me and have supported my efforts with BalleCore over the years and throughout this book-writing process.

First of all, I want to thank all of my former private Pilates and BalleCore clients and students who came to my former studio and allowed me the opportunity to explore, refine, and educate their bodies through developing BalleCore. In particular, I am grateful to Caterina Bandini, a news anchor and reporter, and one of my regular students. She experienced firsthand BalleCore's physical and mental benefits, and was the first to heighten the program's visibility in her capacity as a reporter. I am also appreciative to my loyal students at The Sports Club/LA in Boston who continue to inspire me by coming to class consistently and always staying focused and positive.

A very warm thank-you to my former teachers from whom over the years I have learned a great deal. Special thanks to Martha Mason, Juanita Lopez, Romana Kryzanowska, and Sheri Senese.

Thank you Jacquelyn Stathis at The Sports Club/LA for being the first to offer BalleCore at such a respected health and fitness club, and for your continued support. Michele Hanlon, group exercise manager at Equinox, and Tracie

Finan, creative program director at Healthworks Fitness Centers for Women, have been such passionate supporters of BalleCore, which has been instrumental to the program's success. Thank you, Carol Scott; as director of ECA World Fitness and as a respected fitness professional, your recognition of BalleCore as an innovative fitness program opened many doors.

I am grateful to Laura Young, Principal at the Boston Ballet, for giving me the opportunity not only to teach Pilates but the chance to introduce my program to the school's young dancers. It's been such a privilege to teach Pilates and BalleCore at the Ballet these many years.

Thank you to the dedicated BalleCore instructors whom I have trained, and who are now teaching BalleCore all over the world. Your zeal to teach BalleCore and your hard work does not go unnoticed. You are reaching out to so many people who are looking for an elegant and smart way to exercise! Special thanks to my first BalleCore instructor and good friend, Nancy Jesson, who is always supportive, and to my first Teacher Trainer, Cristina Bruno of Bodywork in Westport, Connecticut; your loyalty to me and BalleCore, your knowledge of movement and creative energy is appreciated. Also, thank you to my colleague Nora Gomez-Dears, whose special lectures have inspired many instructors in my training program. To my West Coast instructors, Charlyn Huss d'Anconia of Core Body Knowledge, thank you for coordinating efforts to establish BalleCore in California, and to Dawn-Marie Ickes, of Core Conditioning in Studio City, California, whose educational feedback and support for BalleCore has been extremely helpful. To Luis Bravo, BalleCore instructor and Web designer, your patience and artistic ability is greatly appreciated.

Thanks to Nina Marquis, MD, for providing BalleCore's first medical endorsement and for offering insightful feedback on improving the program. You've been a loyal student and friend who recognized all the program's potential from the beginning.

Elizabeth Moon, makeup artist, thank you for making me look good during the long photo shoots. You managed to keep me looking fresh all day, and your positive attitude and laughter were just what I needed! Thank you for being a loyal student, too. Thank you Cristine Wu at Lord's & Lady's for doing a great job with my hair—you miraculously kept each strand in place through every exercise. Ted Lopes, owner and trainer of Innovative Fitness, thank you for helping me feel centered and strong for the photo shoot.

Karl Aspelund, thank you for your unique and professional illustrations. I appreciate your attention to detail and for working at such a fast pace. Thank you, Jennifer, for leading the right illustrator in my direction.

Angela Sterling, thank you for your incredible photography and for making this book the best it could be. Your love of movement and photography is so evident. It was such a pleasure to work with you, and thank you for going above and beyond.

Also, Ben, thank you for your assistance in the final hours. Your knowledge of computers and photography was a huge help with getting the right files to the right people at Ballantine.

I am extremely grateful to my literary agent, Laurie Abkemeier at DeFiore and Company, for her ongoing guidance from the very beginning. You have made this process an enjoyable and unforgettable experience. My thanks also to Brian DeFiore for providing his valuable expertise.

Tricia Woods of Sparkatects Inc., thank you for always supporting my goals with BalleCore. You have been instrumental in making my vision with BalleCore become a reality. Your marketing knowledge, professionalism, and ongoing support will always be valued.

To all the people at Ballantine, Johanna Bowman, editorial assistant; Vincent La Scala, production editor; Stacy Rockwood-Chen, production manager; Laura Jorstad, copy editor; Beth Tondreau and Suzanne Dell'Orto, designers; and Sarina Evan, publicist, my enduring thanks for all of your hard work. Special thanks to Maureen O'Neal, editorial director, who led the book production process from start to finish with never-ending enthusiasm. I am honored to have had the opportunity to write this book with such a dynamic team of professionals.

I would like to thank my family and close friends for always listening, and for truly being happy for me and my accomplishments.

Last, if it weren't for the love, patience, and ongoing support of my husband, BalleCore would not have evolved. Thank you so much, Jack, and to my little girls, Elisabeth and Olivia, you have brought tremendous joy to my life!

CONTENTS

FOREWORD

I have learned from years in the medical profession that good health, longevity, and mind–body wellness result from more than just good medicine. In a world where stress, busy schedules, and chronic preventable illnesses are commonplace, it is vital to bring more wellness into our lives by complementing the best of what modern medicine has to offer. Fortunately, Molly Weeks has developed and introduced the BalleCore Workout to fill this great need.

BalleCore is an ideal program for optimizing mind and body capacity. Through movements enhancing balance, precision, and creativity, BalleCore unleashes innate healing powers from within. The program is revolutionary in that it maintains the integrity of the classical arts of ballet, hatha yoga, and Pilates while making them physiologically sound and accessible to everyone. Molly Weeks has brilliantly paired inspiring music to a flow of movements that feel like the playing and dancing long forgotten since childhood. In this place of freedom, fun, flexibility, and grace, participants get in touch with their bodies and the many ways the body and mind are able and meant to function.

Body awareness, highly regarded in Eastern philosophy and culture, is the first step to mind–body wellness and good self-care, and BalleCore opens the door to this healthy path of discovery and health. In Western culture, freedom of expression and compassion toward oneself are often sacrificed for achievement and material pursuits. As a result, stress often takes its toll on the body and mind in the form of joint ailments, obesity, heart disease, anxiety, and depression, to name just a few. To prevent and ameliorate some of these chronic conditions, BalleCore is a perfect outlet with its emphasis on flexibility, balance, and core strength, which all help prevent injury, reduce stress, and increase body focus and awareness.

The creative expression, enjoyment, and poise that come from experiencing BalleCore are additional powerful benefits that enhance emotional well-being, prevent anxiety and depression, and can lead to a more fulfilling life. A healthy frame of mind and sense of freedom lead to inner calm, confidence, and optimism.

Weeks's inspiring teaching creates a delightful, accessible, and safe environment for people of all ages and fitness levels. Her program is as well suited for the first-time exerciser as it is for trained dancers who desire to incorporate elements of other classical movement arts, freedom of expression, and fun into their overall fitness regimen. There is no doubt in my mind that BalleCore can be an invaluable program for anybody seeking mind–body wellness, longevity, and overall good health.

—NINA MARQUIS, MD, MS
physician, wellness coach, and co-founder of Adara

The BalleCore® Workout

INTRODUCTION

I have been involved in some sort of physical activity—whether playing a sport, or taking aerobics or dance classes—since I was a child. Looking back, I didn't have the worries then that I have today. Staying fit and dealing with stress weren't issues. When I reached my 20s and began to work, however, I found that the time I once had to enjoy my favorite physical activities was becoming increasingly difficult to manage. Running to a ballet or jazz class seemed to be more hassle than it was worth, and not being able to attend regularly made class feel more intimidating. I never really liked jogging, but I would force myself to go a mile or two now and then just to get the cardiovascular benefits. As for group exercise, no particular class inspired me enough to want to stick with it. I found myself taking "a little of this and a little of that" and juggling the aerobic-studio and dance-studio schedules for nearly a decade. By the time I reached my late 20s, my motivation to exercise regularly—and my ability to take pleasure in it—had nearly vanished.

Then, in 1996, I was preparing to start a new life with my husband-to-be. I was looking for a change, and wanted to find a career that I could connect with personally as well as professionally. I had taken my first Pilates workshop in Chicago—a rarity at the time—with Juanita Lopez, the only instructor in the Midwest certified to teach the Pilates Method. I began to read article after article about the rebirth of Pilates, and after experiencing it firsthand, I became very inspired. Shortly after, I decided to enroll in a Pilates instructor training program under the tutelage of master trainer Romana Kryzanowska, Joseph Pilates's protégée, and her student Juanita Lopez.

During this time, I was still working full time for the city of Chicago, taking private Pilates lessons and learning how to teach the method to others, as well as trying to keep up with my dance classes. The studio where I was studying ballet at the time, The Conservatory of Dance, offered a ballet/calisthenics class that was fun- and movement-oriented. The director, Sheri Senese, was the first person I know of to bring together performance, beauty and integrity in a mat workout. The music and fluid movements made it easy to stay motivated, but it was not a class for beginners. It was my first glimpse of what a truly beautiful workout class could feel like, and it motivated me to find a way to bring that beauty into a more accessible workout. It was Sheri's classes that got me thinking about how to create my own formula that included the elements of not just ballet, but also Pilates and yoga, as one. I recognized early on the benefits of all three.

Moving to Boston, getting married, and becoming acclimated to my new life gave me time to reflect on what I wanted to get out of Pilates. I continued to work with many teachers throughout New England and found that there was more than one interpretation of Pilates. After I received my certification from the Physicalmind Institute, I decided to open a small, intimate studio, where I taught Pilates to men and women of all ages.

Pilates allowed my clients to feel better while exercising, and it improved their body awareness. Their aches and pains diminished. Many learned to focus inward and were soon open to trying new exercises. Before long, I realized that learning and teaching Pilates was only the beginning of my journey.

I began bringing students to the ballet barre and introduced basic ballet at the end of my Pilates classes. For some, it was very new; for others it brought back wonderful memories. After numerous requests, I started offering ballet and yoga classes. To spice up my Pilates classes, I began deviating from the traditional sequence I had learned and introducing more ballet and yoga movements into the routine. Traditionally, Pilates and yoga classes do not use music during a session, but I always had light classical music playing. Clients liked it so much, they began bringing their own music to share.

I continued to teach at my studio, and I also began teaching at the Boston Ballet. But I found myself spending more time researching and testing the initial BalleCore classes at local dance studios, health clubs, universities, and community centers in order to receive feedback and further refine the program. The dance studios were the first to offer BalleCore to their clients, but I knew that I wanted to reach out to the nondancer as well. I wanted to bring ballet, Pilates, and yoga to people of every age, every fitness level. In my heart, I believed that I could create a perfect program—one that would be accessible and creative for the novice while still challenging for the expert fitness enthusiast.

Guided by my intuition and extensive work with clients, I learned that ballet, Pilates, and yoga are very accessible to everyone when presented in the right environment. The atmosphere has to be nurturing, safe, and inviting. So for the next few years (and two pregnancies!), I worked to fine-tune my own technique and perfect the BalleCore Workout.

The program can be broken into two separate workouts. The first portion (30 minutes in duration) involves mat work, which strengthens and stretches the major muscles and joints, activates the core, mobilizes the spine, and energizes the body. The second portion (20 minutes) involves standing exercises to test balance, coordination, stamina, and full body control.

BalleCore requires you to concentrate completely on the body so that you can move as a unified whole. This is a purposeful workout. No exercise is boring or repetitive. Quite the contrary: The movements require focus, fluidity, and attention to form. The entire body is worked from head to toe. Your mind and body will feel reconnected, and you will be inspired.

The Three Pillars of BalleCore

I chose Pilates, classical ballet, and hatha yoga as the three pillars of BalleCore primarily because they are tried-and-true disciplines. They have been around forever for the right reasons. They are not fads or quick fixes. Nor are they boring. All three methods are elegant ways to achieve a high level of fitness.

But who has time to devote three or more hours a week to a ballet class, a yoga class, *and* a Pilates class? When I created BalleCore, I combined the best elements of each discipline and put an end to the running around.

Here is a thumbnail look at their histories and what each contributes to the BalleCore Workout.

Pilates

The Pilates method of body conditioning is a unique system of stretching and strengthening exercises developed more than 90 years ago by Joseph H. Pilates. Pilates began developing his system in Germany in the early 1900s. He was a weak child who was determined to strengthen his body through exercise. He studied the body and became proficient in skiing, boxing, gymnastics, and bodybuilding. While he was detained with other prisoners of war in England during World War I, he created exercises to aid in the rehabilitation of prisoners. When he returned home, the German army recognized the importance of his teaching, but because of political pressures Pilates chose not to work for the army after the war. Instead, he immigrated to the United States and settled in New York City.

Before his method was called Pilates, Joseph H. Pilates himself named it Contrology. His method reinforced full body control, focus, and quality, rather than mindless repetition and quantity. He fused Eastern and Western beliefs while focusing on strengthening and stretching the whole body. He also emphasized the core or "powerhouse" of the body. And his theory proves to be popular today. Joseph H. Pilates believed that a strong and supple back and a powerful center are requisites for a healthy body.

BalleCore incorporates the fundamentals of Pilates to take advantage of the countless benefits of a core-conditioning workout. Strengthening the core helps improve balance, which is so important as we get older. Believe it or not, balance degeneration starts at age 25. And for women already challenged by the threat of osteoporosis, loss of balance can mean more injuries from falling. Working the core also helps strengthen posture. Great posture is key to those who have to work long days at a desk or in front of a computer. Not only do you look better with shoulders back and stomach in, but you feel added energy as breathing becomes more natural. It also reduces backaches and muscle stress.

Hatha Yoga

There are many types of yoga—Iyengar, Ashtanga, and vinyasa, to name just a few. I selected my favorite foundational hatha yoga postures to incorporate into the BalleCore program because they are considered universal exercises.

Hatha yoga is the world's most ancient mind–body practice. *Hatha* literally means "union of sun and moon"—in essence, the union of body and mind, emotion and spirit. Hatha yoga consists of a series of physical postures, or asanas. Through a sequence of asanas, we learn to quiet the mind by placing focus on the breath, or pranayama, and by connecting breath to movement. Yoga philosophy regards the body as the temple of the divine spirit, which should therefore be cared for and appreciated as a temple.

Many people are first drawn to yoga as a way to keep fit, but, depending on your desire and discipline, it can be much more than physical exercise. Yoga tones the internal organs, regulates the hormones, strengthens the nervous system, builds a strong and flexible muscular physique, and produces mental equilibrium. Awareness, concentration, and meditation are cultivated through regular practice. This new presence of mind can further help you tap into the present moment, allowing you to overcome fear and redirect behavior patterns successfully.

In BalleCore, we incorporate postures that we may hold for several breaths, more often, we link the postures together, vinyasa style, in a flowing sequence. The BalleCore program teaches you the skills to build a balanced structural base so that each and every yoga position can be accomplished with great strength and pride.

Ballet

The word *ballet* refers to a specific dance technique that was first developed in the late 17th century in France. Some ballet performances tell a story, while others are abstract and present different techniques of dance. All dancers communicate artistically through movement and music during their performance. To watch a ballet is to witness the physical acumen in addition to the artistic qualities of the performers.

Professional dancers need to practice posture, balance, and speed. They work on this during their daily ballet class. Like Pilates and the foundational asanas of yoga, ballet has a set of basic movements, including warm-ups to increase the blood flow to the muscles, and exercises to strengthen the body. The ballet barre used during their daily sessions supports the dancers as they perform the exercises. These exercises prepare the dancers for more advanced movements without the barre, when good balance and spatial awareness are needed.

In BalleCore, I have incorporated classical ballet movements such as the relevé (raising the heels) and plié (bending the knees). The workout also uses an optional freestanding apparatus called the BalleCore Barre, which is similar to a ballet barre. The BalleCore Barre helps promote good posture, core stability, and balance while you perform standing work and mat work.

A Powerful Combination

To be good at any sport or hobby, a clear mind is paramount. Pilates, yoga, and ballet all require focus and *mindfulness*. BalleCore uses fundamental techniques designed to draw you in: proper breathing, complete concentration, deliberate movements, and attention to precision and control.

Pilates, ballet, and yoga complement one another so well, not only because they require a brain–body connection, but also because together they create a well-balanced, challenging, and creative workout. All three modes of exercise require the strengthening and lengthening of muscles, focused breathing, and facilitating power from the core. The BalleCore Workout challenges you further by blending balance training with dynamic movement. I have chosen an array of effective and approachable exercises from the three disciplines and created variations to make them safe and enjoyable. Combined with signature BalleCore, these exercises will prepare you for a delightful way to move through life. You will experience inner calm and increased body awareness while receiving all the physical benefits as well.

Equally important, you will not only feel the benefits, but also see results. Your posture will become better as you develop an awareness of working the body as a whole rather than working isolated muscles. Your arms, legs, and core will become stronger and more sculpted, looking trimmer than ever. Areas that were once tight and stiff will open up as you gain incredible ease throughout your body as you move in many directions. You will reduce stress and feel better about tackling your everyday hurdles. We all have them, but when we are balanced and in control, we discover we can make the right decisions. Most of all, you will have a better appreciation of who you are and what you want to accomplish on your journey to optimal health and longevity.

BalleCore allows you the opportunity to express your creativity and challenge yourself in the privacy of your own home. It is the next step toward staying healthy, feeling motivated, and achieving a state of grace while exercising. Why grunt and groan through a workout when you can be graceful instead? With this routine, guaranteed, you will feel beautiful.

So let's get started!

GETTING STARTED

BalleCore is a beautiful way to exercise the mind and body. It is a thoughtful technique that requires you to be conscious of what is happening with your body inside and out. In this chapter, you will learn all the elements—including the six BalleCore Foundations and the five Body Concepts—that are necessary for you to exercise attentively and truly enjoy it. They are easy to follow and will guide you all the way.

BalleCore Foundations

Physical stress and mental anxiety are common obstacles in today's world. When was the last time you found the time to relax and focus on fully inhaling and exhaling? It isn't always easy to do. We all have busy schedules, and thinking about past events or your "to do" list isn't the best way to initiate an exercise program. First and foremost, you need to feel comfortable and create your own atmosphere—one that allows you to tune in. Staying focused and relaxed sets the stage for a more pleasurable workout, and you will find that you become naturally drawn in. Take the following steps to begin your workout.

Relax Your Body and Mind

We have become conditioned to tense up, hold our breath, and strain muscles. Freeing your mind and oxygenating the muscles before you begin the program will help disentangle and release tense areas in the body, providing a more enjoyable experience for you. A relaxed, full breath enhances mindfulness during your daily life and while working out. When you are ready to start the BalleCore program, relax to release tension, but remember to maintain tone and control throughout the body. At first, you'll need to remind yourself that you are actually sitting still, breathing, and staying in the moment. But with practice, it will come naturally.

1. Prepare by either lying down or sitting in the tailor's seat position (cross-legged).
2. Clear your mind by bringing attention to your breath.
3. Close your eyes and inhale slowly. Feel your lungs and belly expand. Slowly exhale.
4. Bring attention to your muscles and relax every muscle in the body.
5. Slowly scan your body from your toes to the crown of your head.
6. Let go of any negative or stressful thoughts about the day.

Breathe

When breath stops, so does flow! Breathing disentangles and releases tense areas in the body. Breathing with attention can help you during exercise and your daily life. A relaxed, full breath enhances mindfulness. Remember, you are using breath and exercise to create equilibrium in the body.

The BalleCore breathing technique is designed to work with each exercise. It will improve the quality of how you move and how you feel. And it will strengthen your deep abdominal muscles and lower back, which is essential for the BalleCore routine.

The BalleCore Breathing Technique

1. Tailor-sit, lifting off your sitting bones.

2. Lift your abdominal muscles in and up, creating length from your hips to ribs.
3. Lengthen the base of your torso.
4. With your elbows pointing out to the sides, place your hands on your ribs, spreading your fingers.
5. Slowly inhale through your nose. Feel the rib cage expand to the sides and into your back as your diaphragm descends.
6. Exhale slowly and completely through your mouth, drawing your belly toward your spine and feeling your ribs knit together.

Exhaling completely gets you in touch with your deepest muscles. Focused breathing also keeps the muscles warm, causing them to lengthen and open up the spaces between each vertebra and rib so that the body expands to create a longer, leaner shape. A basic abdominal contraction occurs with every exhale and is the preparation for each and every exercise. This continuous support must be emphasized at the beginning, middle, and end of an exercise. Always exhale on the muscle contraction or exertion, and inhale on the muscle release and extension. Maintain the lift in your rib cage and keep your neck and throat soft. Keep your shoulder blades down.

Stabilize the Core

Rather than rounding your shoulders and sinking into your hip area with your tummy relaxed, think about creating the longest possible length from head, neck, and upper spine all the way to your tailbone. Now move your attention to your middle.

The band of muscles located in your midsection front and back, from just below your chest to your pubic bone, is called the core. The core is the body's center of power. The deep abdominal muscles that support your pelvis and internal organs (transverse abdominals) and your side muscles (internal and external obliques) stabilize your torso. The surrounding muscle groups, such as the hip, buttocks, and lower back muscles as well as your pelvic floor, need to be strong and flexible in conjunction with your inner core to execute the movements with full control and integrity.

A strong center allows you to move efficiently and become less prone to injury, especially at the joints such as the hips, knees, and ankles. Not only will you find that your sense of balance and muscular control improves by learning to activate your center, but your waistline will appear slimmer, too.

Bring Belly to Back

The action of pulling in your lower abdominal region, specifically your belly button and the area just below, is a good exercise to practice regularly. Whether you are standing, exercising on the mat, or just going about your daily routine, this action will strengthen your lower back and significantly improve your posture. By carefully drawing in your navel and pelvis, you create a flat abdominal wall and lengthen the back. In this position, feel as if you are narrowing your pelvis. This is the point where you want to reinforce a muscle contraction. Always try to lengthen the base of your spine and gently draw the tailbone down toward your heels. Be careful not to suck the stomach in, because it means you are probably holding your breath. You want to maintain an "anchoring" feeling while breathing normally.

If you connect your belly to your back, the BalleCore movements will feel more natural. As you learn the BalleCore routine, you will feel your body moving in many directions. Our bodies have the mobility to move in three dimensions. We will learn exercises that take you forward (flexion), open you up (extension), as well as bending you sideways and spiraling. Moving with good support is an essential part of BalleCore. Follow these steps before moving in any direction.

1. Breathe mindfully.
2. Starting at your navel, draw your abdominal muscles (just below the navel) up and inward.
3. Continue breathing and move your attention to your sides and around to the back.

4. Feel as if your connection is one continuous circle around the waist, remembering that your goal is to establish a strong structural base.

5. Now imagine that you are shrinking this continuous circle, as if you're squeezing out a sponge. This is the point where you want to reinforce a muscle contraction.

6. Inhale, lift up, and notice the lengthening in the spine. Exhale.

Focus

Each movement in BalleCore has a purpose. Some exercises are easier than others, but the same mental focus is required for each. Understand that you are an entity—body, mind, and spirit working in tandem. Although some movements may require more work in one specific muscle group, remember that all of your power initiates from your center. (Think of your belly button as the ignition button.) You will discover that even with the simplest of exercises, your mind needs the same degree of focus as with the more challenging movements.

Be Efficient and Strive for Quality

The quality of movement—doing it right—is more important than the repetition of mindless exercise. Remember, building a strong foundation before you begin your workout is the key. Once you have established a strong center and a conscious breathing technique, you will be ready to move effectively and efficiently.

How you move determines the visible results in your body. If you force an exercise by jerking or moving too quickly without really thinking about the action, you can cause wear and tear on a joint and experience pain. There is no need to waste precious physical and mental energy on thoughtless movements, instead, strive for efficient, continuous, and fluid movements that call for precision, integrity, and grace.

BalleCore Body Concepts

As you work through the exercises, concentrate on which muscles are working and on your overall body position. When your posture is correct, your brain has the ability to better perceive and coordinate movement. Whether you are performing the floor exercises or standing moves, it is imperative to weave together both the Foundations previously discussed and the Body Concepts outlined below.

The Body Concepts will guide you to proper placement while working on the mat or while standing. Each Concept has a function and is part of the overall plan to generate healthy movement from the bones to the joints and out through the muscles.

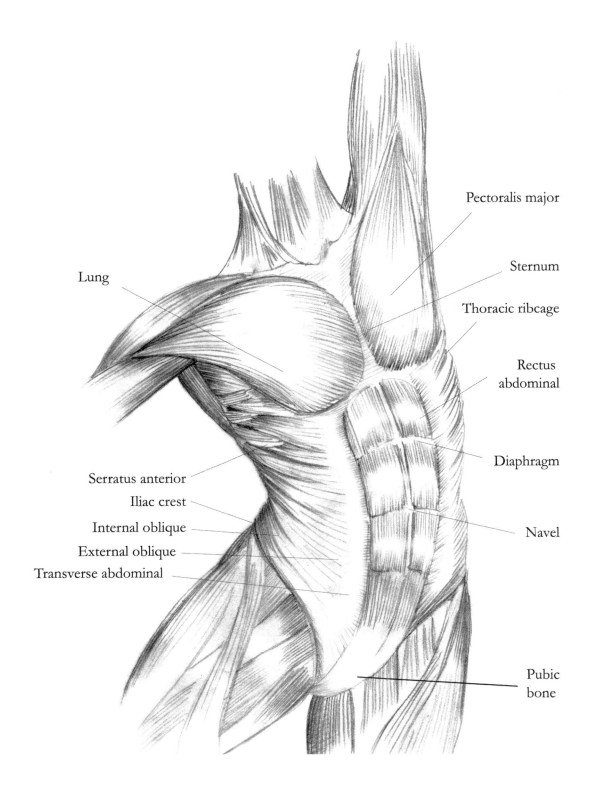

Pectoralis major

Sternum

Thoracic ribcage

Rectus
abdominal

Lung

Diaphragm

Navel

Serratus anterior

Iliac crest

Internal oblique

External oblique

Transverse abdominal

Pubic
bone

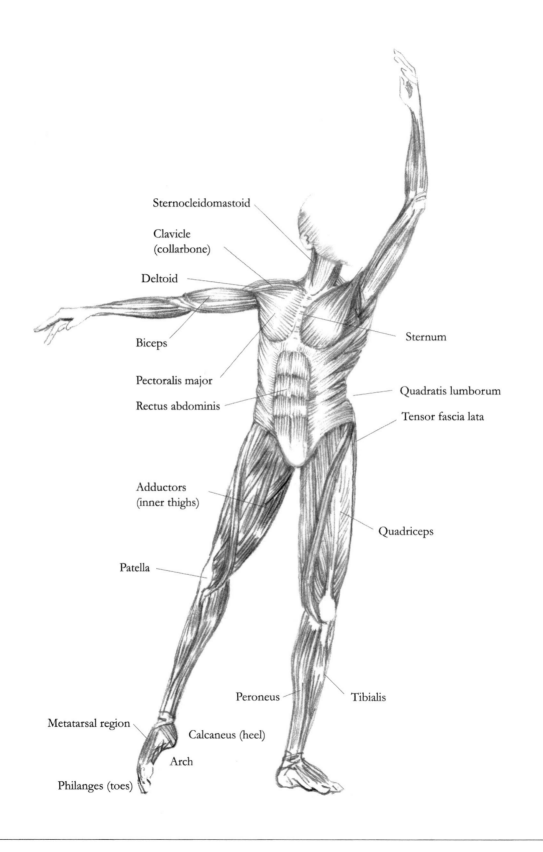

Sternocleidomastoid

Clavicle
(collarbone)

Deltoid

Biceps

Pectoralis major

Rectus abdominis

Adductors
(inner thighs)

Patella

Metatarsal region

Philanges (toes)

Arch

Calcaneus (heel)

Sternum

Quadratis lumborum

Tensor fascia lata

Quadriceps

Peroneus

Tibialis

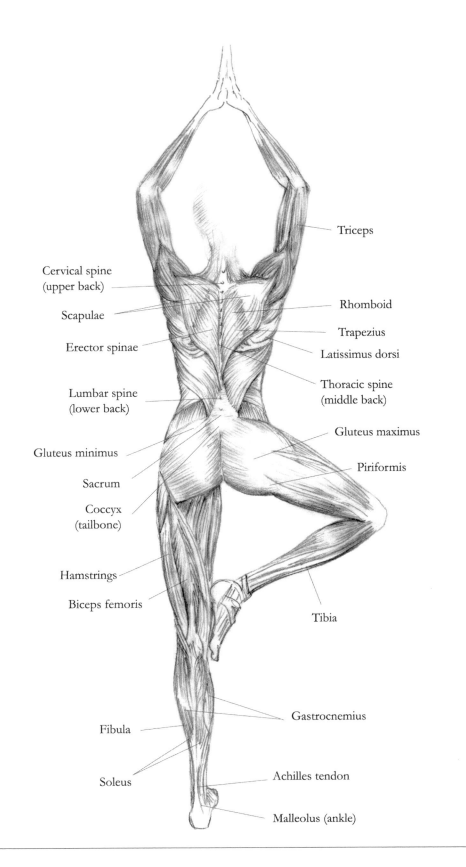

Triceps

Cervical spine
(upper back)

Scapulae

Erector spinae

Lumbar spine
(lower back)

Gluteus minimus

Sacrum

Coccyx
(tailbone)

Hamstrings

Biceps femoris

Fibula

Soleus

Rhomboid

Trapezius

Latissimus dorsi

Thoracic spine
(middle back)

Gluteus maximus

Piriformis

Tibia

Gastrocnemius

Achilles tendon

Malleolus (ankle)

The Neck

The BalleCore Workout works the body from top to toes, starting with gentle body-awakening stretches at the neck and shoulder area. The seven cervical vertebrae are very fragile. While standing, imagine that you are increasing the length from the crown of your head to your tailbone. While lying on the mat, keep your neck long by gently lengthening the back of the neck on the mat as you slightly tuck your chin. Always keep in mind that these vertebrae are part of your spine. During the routine, you'll work to increase the range of motion in your neck, which will in turn make the abdominal exercises more comfortable.

The Shoulders

Tension in the shoulders is a common problem with many of us. Sitting at a computer or talking on the phone while performing another task lends itself to more misalignment in the body. If your shoulders are rounded and tight, the strain will eventually radiate to your neck or other parts of the body. You probably are not thinking about correct posture, but it's only a matter of time before you feel the strain somewhere else.

To correct this problem, in a seated position, pull up out of the waist again by engaging your core muscles, and create length from the tail to the crown of the head. Slide your shoulder blades, or scapulae, down the back toward the lower spine, creating a V. Feel as if the space between the shoulders and chest is opening up wider and wider. Try to avoid pinching the shoulder blades together by opening up too much.

Good range of motion in the shoulder girdle is essential for many of our daily movements as well as with the BalleCore routine. You will feel more open and will be able to accomplish the exercises with more ease and fluidity.

The Pelvis

The BalleCore routine concentrates on stretching and strengthening the front, sides, and back of the hips, as well as the attached muscles such as the spine, buttocks and leg muscles. Optimal strength and flexibility in the hips are essential for pain-free movement during exercise and daily living. Leading a mostly sedentary life or playing a sport that overuses certain muscles can cause both stiffness and imbalance in the hips, which can have adverse effects in other areas of the body such as the spine, legs, and feet. I will show you wonderful exercises to open up your hips and increase your range of motion, making exercise more enjoyable. More important, your chance for an injury or a fall will diminish as you achieve a strong and healthy body.

Practice rotating your pelvis between a posterior tilt (or tucking,) which creates a flat low back, and an anterior tilt (or arching,) which creates excessive space in the low back. To do this, lie down using the floor as a gauge, or turn your body sideways and stand using a mirror to guide you.

1. First, squeeze your buttocks muscles so that your back flattens. Notice how your body feels and what happens to your posture.
2. Now arch the back as if you are sticking out your rear and letting your belly tip forward. If you look at your posture, it may appear a little off, and your lower back may tense up.
3. To align your hips and pelvis correctly, place your hands on your hip bones and draw the tailbone down as you gently lift the abdominal muscles in toward your back. Your pelvis and hip bones should feel lengthened and more even.

This is your starting point and base for all movement. Many muscles attach to the pelvis, and for this reason the position needs to be practiced correctly. When your pelvis is aligned, your spine will be long and your neck and shoulder area will be balanced over your hips.

The Arms and Legs

Do not lock your knees or your elbows. Hyperextending the joints places undue stress on your body. For example, if you place too much pressure on your wrists in a tabletop position (on your hands and knees), you will not be able to sustain the position. First, focus on using the strength and power from your core—this will reduce the likelihood of sinking unnecessary weight into the joints. Second, use the strength of your arms to support your body and help take pressure off your wrists. Also, as you connect with your breathing, your limbs will feel free, allowing your movement to be less controlling and more energetic.

While you are exercising, imagine that you are being stretched out horizontally and vertically, creating length in your legs and arms and away from your center. As you channel this core energy away and out through your limbs, remember to bring it back to your center, staying connected.

The Feet

The placement of your feet is important. As with the pelvis and hips, your feet play a vital role in establishing a strong foundation, which gives you more control. The BalleCore Workout doesn't overlook the importance of proper placement, which strengthens your feet and increases joint motion. Your feet are the foundation and support for your legs. By reinforcing proper alignment with movement integrity, improvements in overall balance and body awareness result. If you often wear high heels or flat shoes, you may experience discomfort and cramping in the calves. BalleCore incorporates relaxing stretches to relieve aches, as well as strengthening exercises to reinforce both your ankles and the muscles and tendons in the bottoms of your feet, your calves, and your inner thighs.

Your feet can be worked in a flexed, half-pointed, or pointed position, or simply relaxed.

1. While standing, feel the weight evenly spread between the balls and the heels of your feet. Practice finding this balance by rocking back and forth.
2. Now, lift your toes and press your heels firmly into the floor.
3. Lift your arch as you spread your toes back onto the floor to widen your base of support.

Other BalleCore exercises are performed with heels lifted. During these moves, maintain weight primarily on the ball area of your big and second toes. Between your second and third toes begin the line of symmetry up to your knees, hips, and shoulders. The connection of your baby toes to the floor assists with basic balance.

With many of the ballet- and Pilates-inspired exercises, your feet need to be fully stretched. Sending breath and energy out through the feet creates a long and lean look, similar to that of a dancer. Tensed toes can cause cramps, so try to spread you toes and "glue" them to the floor. Using the floor to ground you will help with overall balance. Working on your stance consistently will improve coordination, full body control, and awareness of proper body positioning.

Check Back Often

Revisiting the Foundations and Body Concepts regularly will help you improve your structure each time you do the BalleCore Workout. You will notice dramatic results in your hips, thighs, and buttocks, and target your body's deeper muscles. Your motivation to exercise will increase because you will discover new moves that are inspiring and actually feel good. You will learn to let go of the muscle tension that may affect your ability to perform the exercises correctly, while you improve your overall posture and physique.

Precautions

I guarantee that BalleCore can benefit all ages and body types. This doesn't mean that every exercise is appropriate for you all the time, however. We all have limitations and days when our bodies feel tense and stiff. There is no reason to place undue pressure on yourself as you learn the BalleCore Workout. Your first priority is to listen to your own body and observe the sensations in your muscles. Preventing injury and ensuring a safe atmosphere will help you stick with the BalleCore routine. If you need to take it slow or you're not feeling 100 percent, BalleCore includes superb gentler exercises and stretches to prepare you for the more vigorous work to follow.

If you are a beginner and would like to approach BalleCore with more ease the first few times around, you should start with the BalleCore Express or other Time-Saver programs found on page 249. These programs are shorter versions of the complete 50-minute routine. Once you gain a solid understanding of the Body Concepts and Foundations, your focus will gradually increase while your muscles' memory improves. Strain is less likely to happen with increased concentration.

You will come back to BalleCore time after time because of its emphasis on working at your own level and tuning into your own body. For instance, if you have little or no Pilates training, you may decide to keep your head on the floor for some of the abdominal work. If coordination isn't easy, such as moving the arms and legs simultaneously, you may choose to leave out the BalleCore Barre and modify the exercise. BalleCore allows you to take the next step at any time in the workout.

Here are a few guidelines to keep in mind:

- If a certain exercise is putting strain on an area in your body, stop and reread the instructions or follow the recommended modification. Remember to breathe and apply the BalleCore Foundations. This will guide you to correct muscle usage and positive results.
- If you experience specific discomfort in your lower back or neck area due to a position or movement that doesn't feel right, I have two important rules. First, immediately lower your head. Take a breath in and rest for a moment. If the problem continues, place a small pillow or towel under your head and continue to exercise. Second, for relief

in the back, simply bend the knees and bring the feet to the floor to release the lumbar vertebrae in the lower spine.

- If you are pregnant, follow the American College of Obstetricians and Gynecologists (ACOG) guidelines and consult your health practitioner. Many of the positions are not appropriate for pregnancy, which is why many dance and fitness studios offer a Prenatal BalleCore program tailored specifically for pregnant women. Still, the BalleCore Workout is a great way to get in shape and increase your energy *after* the birth of a baby.

Uniquely BalleCore

There are two components of the BalleCore Workout that are unique to BalleCore: a portable ballet barre and the use of motivational music. Although neither of these is required to reap the benefits of the program, both will enhance your enjoyment and increase the likelihood that you will stick with it.

The BalleCore Barre

In the classroom setting, I use a beautiful, rock maple, 4-foot barre that has been custom-designed for the BalleCore Workout. It has doughnut-shaped ends that offer additional support and a comfortable position for the hands. Emulating the classical ballet barre that you see in dance studios, the BalleCore Barre is also portable, allowing every participant to progress at his or her own pace. It's a versatile tool that I use for most of the exercises in the BalleCore Workout. While using it on the floor, it helps me to stabilize my upper body and tone my arms and shoulder area. The continuous use of the barre makes the exercises increasingly challenging, sending energy and heat to all the muscles in the body; this speeds up your metabolism and burns fat. It's also a great way to measure range of motion and flexibility. The barre is lightweight, so you can really create resistance with your own body weight.

While standing, in the second half of the workout, the barre is used for dependable support and balance training. Beginners hold on to it with two hands. If you are more experienced, you can hold it at chest level in front of your body, or hold it to the side to free up one arm. The beauty of the barre is its versatility. At any point in the workout, you can alter the position of the barre to suit your fitness level.

You should never use a weighted body bar for BalleCore. The purpose of the barre is not to build muscle or place undue stress on the body, but rather to improve coordination, generate body heat, develop greater agility, and strengthen your core.

The Music

The classroom version of the BalleCore Workout is choreographed to music. Good music can move you or relax you. For many, it is also a confidence booster—a way to jump-start your self-esteem. Listening to your favorite music will enhance your workout. You'll feel more enthusiastic, and you'll notice a stronger connection between your mind and body as they work together in time with the beat. The music you choose will guide you through a tangible, conscious workout where movements transition from one to the next, leaving you feeling complete. This increased brain–body connection cultivates better balance and a natural fluidity in the body.

We all have different tastes in music. I recommend choosing music that helps you forget about your hectic schedule and draws you into the moment. It will also feel easier to follow the rhythm as you move your body. Your movements will connect more gracefully. Choose your favorite pop singer or tenor and turn up the volume to where you feel completely connected. The beauty of doing this workout in your own space is that it gives you total control over the music.

I recommend different kinds of music, ranging from revamped classical and world music to Brazilian samba, techno, and pop. Keep your workout fresh by experimenting with new music. You will be pleasantly surprised at how easy the exercises become and how creative you'll feel moving to the beat! Here are some of my favorites:

- ARIA, a modern twist to opera arias.
- *Buddha-Bar*, a compilation of inspiring world music.
- Sasha Lazard, a vocalist, combines classical with techno.
- Ottmar Liebert, flamenco guitarist.
- Cirque du Soleil, the international dance troupe.
- Chopin, Ravel, and Vivaldi, classical.
- Madredeus, Portuguese easy listening.
- Tom Jobim, bossa nova.
- Secret Garden, Irish-influenced music featuring violin, piano, harp, and some vocals.
- Maxwell, cool jazz.
- *Visage I* and *Visage II*, compilations of global music with a beat.
- Jewel, a female vocalist—both pop and folk.
- Alessandro Safina, Italian tenor, pop opera.
- Café del Mar, a compilation of eclectic music from around the world.
- Dido, a female vocalist, pop.

What Will I Need to Begin?

To prepare for your BalleCore routine, you will need the following:

✓ **The Right Space:** First, locate a spot where you would like to exercise. Find enough uncluttered space so that you won't feel cramped or interrupted. A carpeted floor is good and can offer more support for your back. For the standing section of the workout, a hardwood or tiled floor is ideal so that your feet don't slip and you can ground yourself.

✓ **Yoga or Exercise Mat:** Yoga mats are very thin and don't necessarily protect and cushion the back, but they are great for preventing your hands and feet from slipping. If you feel you need extra support for the back, then make sure you are working in a carpeted area. A firm exercise mat is fine for the floor work, but it isn't recommended for the standing portion—you may experience slipping.

✓ **Small Pillow or Small Towel**: If you experience neck pain, the support of a pillow or towel will offer relief.

✓ **An Exercise Band Such as a BalleCore Band**: Extra support while stretching helps open up tight muscles and ensure that you are doing the movements correctly. If you experience significant stiffness in the hip or hamstring area, it is easy to fall out of alignment. To help you stay focused on opening up your tight area, a band is preferred. It has more "give" than a yoga strap or tie. It also is a great strengthening tool for your ankles.

✓ **BalleCore Barre, 1 1/4-Inch Dowel or Sturdy Chair**: If you do not have a BalleCore Barre, I recommend an alternative tool for support. A sturdy chair for beginners will guide you during much of the standing work. Once you master the moves and improve balance, an inexpensive 1 1/4-inch dowel from your local hardware store is a good choice. The specific exercises will illustrate how to use the barre or an alternative.

✓ **Inspiring Music**: Select an album at least one hour in duration. Or choose several albums if you have a multi-CD player, and press the "SHUFFLE" button to experience a variety of tunes—different every workout.

✓ **No Interruptions**: Unplug the phone. Turn off your cell phone. This is your time.

What Should I Wear?

When it comes to exercise wear, it really depends on your personal preference. There is so much exercise attire available these days—gym shorts, yoga pants, leggings, leotards . . . choose whatever is most comfortable for you. No footwear is necessary.

When Should I Work Out?

Exercise can be done whenever it fits into your life. Some people prefer to wake up and work out before their day begins, while others make the time after work when their day winds down. Your lifestyle will determine how you approach exercise. If you want to see visible, immediate results, you should do the complete exercise program three times a week and schedule accordingly. Of course, this doesn't mean that you cannot feel or look better by practicing the program once or twice a week! The important thing to remember is to set realistic goals so that you stay motivated. When you choose to make the time to exercise, review the Foundations. They are your guide to exercising in a healthy state of mind. They will prepare you for the exercises to come and ensure that you enjoy what you are doing.

And if time is a concern, don't give up. Skip to the BalleCore Time-Savers and find a specialized program that suits you. If you are busy working long hours or are traveling, BalleCore Express has been designed to keep you motivated and on the right track. But even the complete BalleCore Workout takes less than an hour. No matter what you choose, BalleCore is a time-efficient method of exercising the mind and body. Stick with it!

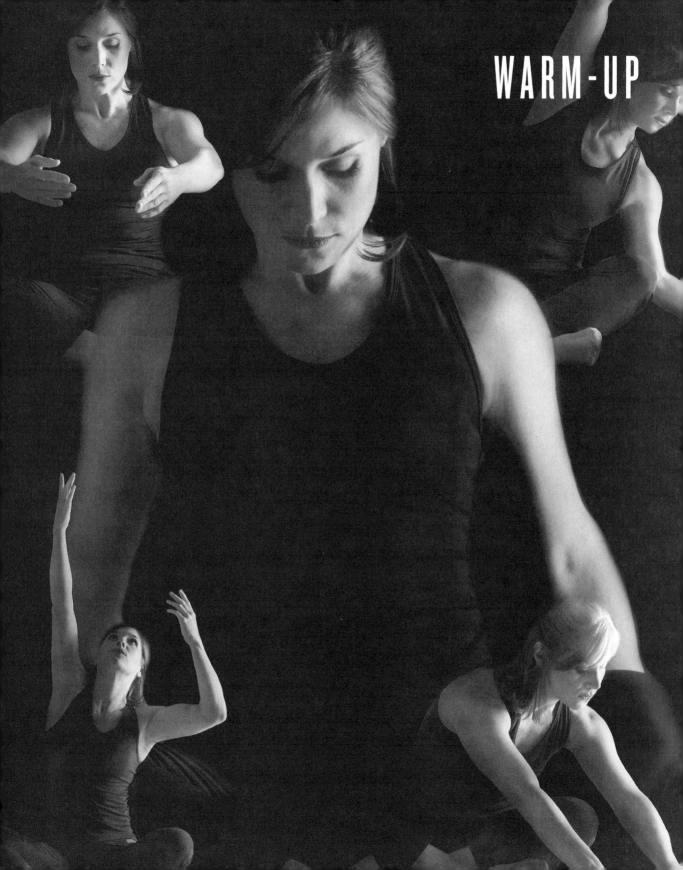

Warm-Up

Each time you start a BalleCore workout, you begin with gentle body-awakening stretches. These stretching movements are an important part of the program and should never be left out of your BalleCore experience. The purpose of warming up is to slowly energize the body, bring awareness to how you breathe, and help you learn to listen to how your body feels prior to moving deeper into the program. You start by releasing tension in the head, neck, and shoulder areas, and complete this section by learning where your center of power is located and understanding how to activate your core. It is during this section that you first connect the body and mind in order to achieve inner relaxation, and learn to exercise with more confidence and control over your body. This warm-up feels great, so relax and enjoy it.

Benefits:

❏ Encourages the muscles to relax and enhances lung capacity.
❏ Replenishes levels of energy as blood circulates to warm muscles.
❏ Brings awareness to your center.

Breathing Exercise

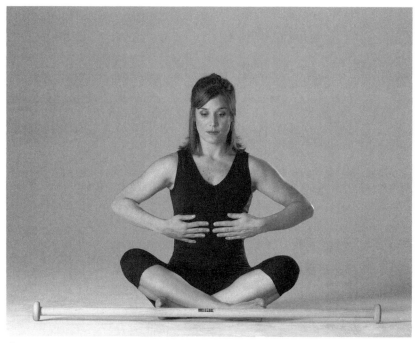

1. Sit cross-legged with your hands on your rib cage and with your elbows wide at your sides. Take a breath in through your nose as you expand your rib cage.

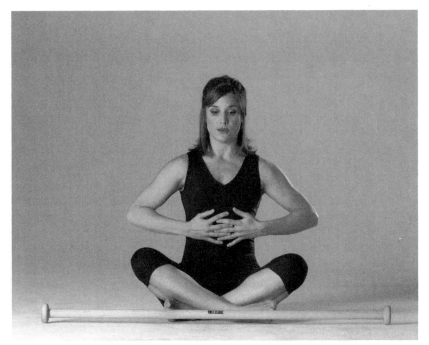

2. Exhale completely out through your mouth as you knit your ribs and fingers together.

REPEAT 3 TIMES

HELPFUL REMINDERS:

- Lift off your seat as you gently squeeze your buttock muscles.

- Press your shoulders down as you lift the sternum.

- Bring your abdominal muscles toward the spine by actively pulling in and up. Narrow your pelvis.

- Maintain control as you breathe naturally, yet mindfully.

Arm Reaches

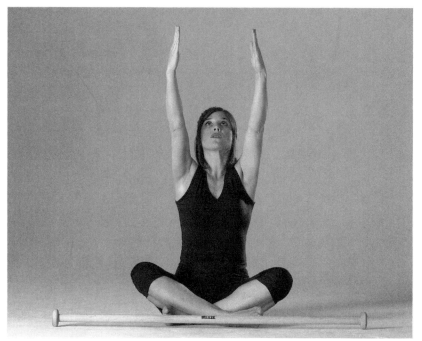

1. Stretch your arms and fingers out to the sides. Inhale, slowly
stretch your arms overhead, and look up.

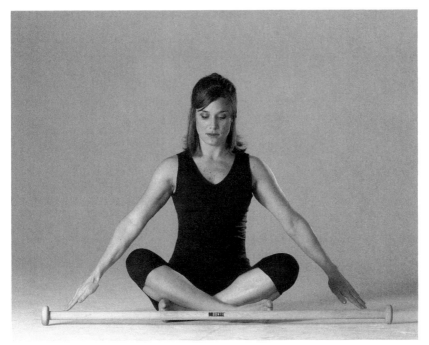

2. Exhale, and lengthen your arms as you lower them to your sides.

REPEAT 3 TIMES

HELPFUL REMINDERS:

- Continue to activate your buttock and abdominal muscles as you move your arms.

- As you bring your arms overhead, the shoulder blades should be drawn down.

Arm Reaches with Forward Bend

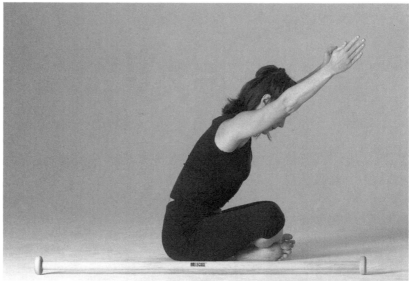

HELPFUL REMINDERS:

- As you bend forward, activate your core and legs so you don't lose control and tip forward.

- Take your time as you roll through your spine, and remember to breathe.

1. Inhale, slowly stretch your arms overhead, and look up. Stretch your arms and torso forward while keeping your back flat. Keep your seat down.

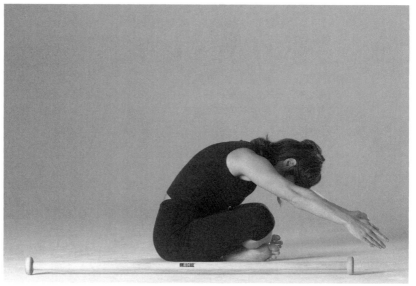

2. Continue bending forward, or cambré forward, and let your upper back and neck stretch. Roll up through the spine one vertebra at a time, starting at your tailbone and finishing at the top of the head.

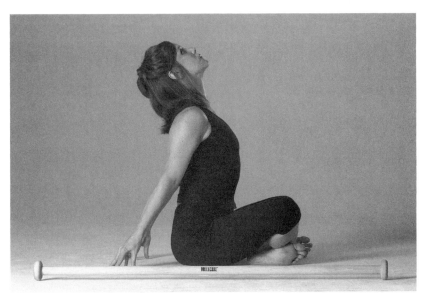

3. Walk your fingers to the back and bring your shoulder blades together, expanding your chest and shoulders. Stretch your neck carefully as you look up.

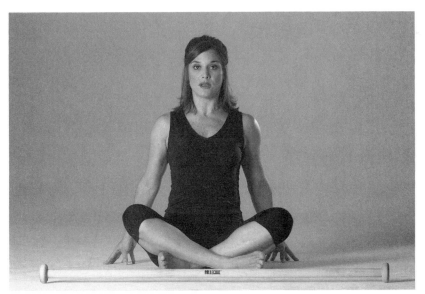

4. Bring your chin and head level and continue to lengthen your back.

REPEAT 3 TIMES

Core Contractions

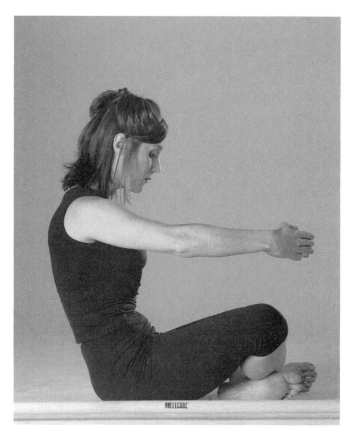

1. Inhale, and stretch your arms out to the sides with your palms facing front. Exhale, and scoop your lower abdominals into your back as you round your arms forward.

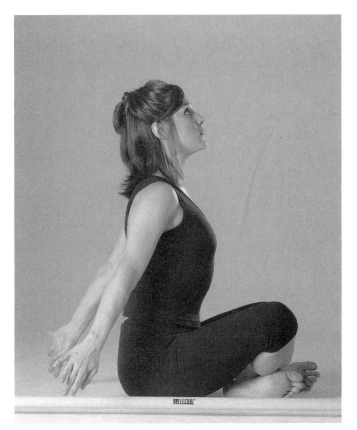

2. Inhale, and press your arms away as you lift your chest and chin.

REPEAT 4 TIMES

HELPFUL REMINDERS:

- To begin, lift up off your seat by activating your buttock muscles.
- Draw your abdominals inward and up before you start scooping, to avoid injuring your lower back and tailbone.

Quarter Turn with Forward Bend

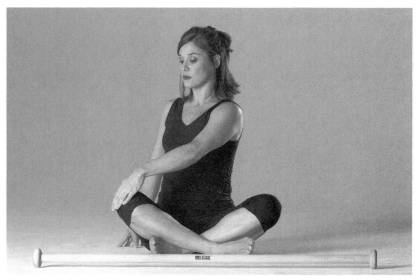

1. Inhale, and rotate your trunk so the opposite shoulder is in line with your knee. Place your hand on your knee to lengthen spine.

HELPFUL REMINDERS:

- To begin, square off your shoulders and hips.

- Lengthen your spine as you rotate the torso and chest to your opposite knee.

- Keep your elbows slightly rounded, and draw the shoulder blades down.

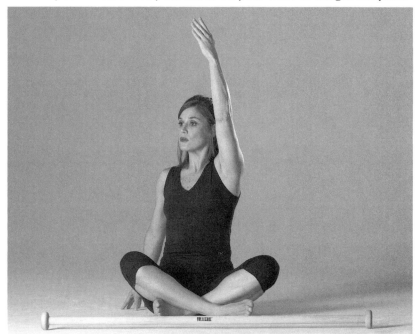

2. Inhale as you raise your arm up to your ear. This is the fifth port de bras position.

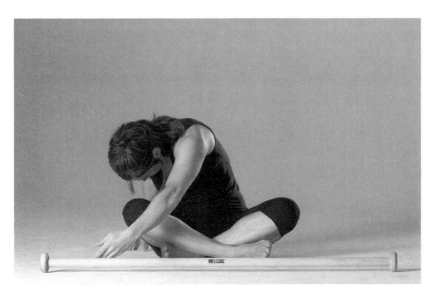

3. Exhale and bend forward, or cambré, to your knee.

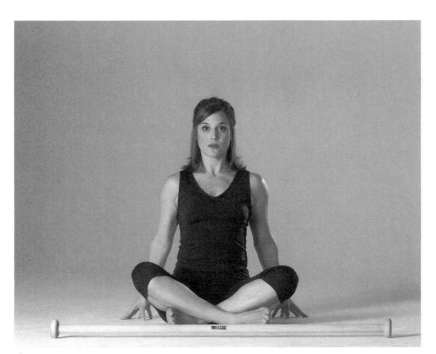

4. Inhale and raise your arm back to your ear to fifth port de bras.
   Exhale and bring your body to face front.

5. Repeat to the other side.

R E P E A T   2   T I M E S

Side Port de Bras

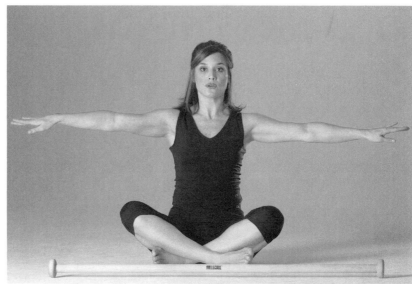

1. Stretch your arms to the side with your palms facing front and your elbows slightly rounded.

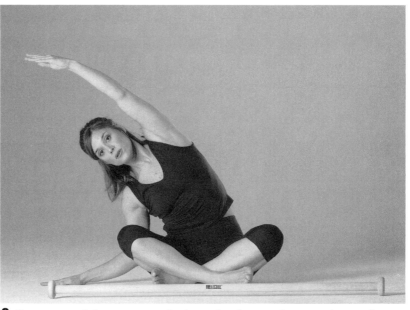

2. Bring your left arm up with the palm facing down and stretch to the side. Press your right hand firmly into floor.

HELPFUL REMINDERS:

- Anchor your seat as you gently squeeze your buttock muscles.

- Press your shoulders down as you lift your arms to the sides and overhead.

- When your arms are stretched at your sides, your fingers should be in your peripheral vision.

- Bring your abdominal muscles toward the spine by actively pulling in and up.

- Stack the ribs as you stretch your torso directly to the side. Keep your hips down.

- Breathe naturally.

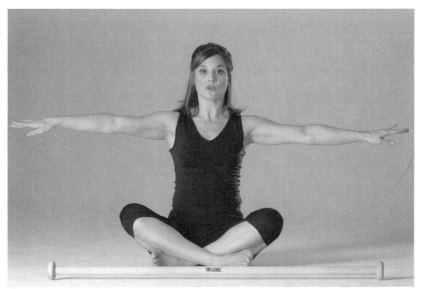

3. Stretch your arms to the side.

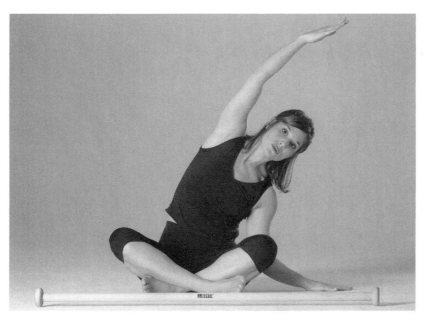

4. Bring your right arm up and stretch to the other side.
Press your left hand into the floor.

5. Finish with both arms stretched to the sides and
touching the floor.

REPEAT 4 TIMES

Roll-Down with Port de Bras

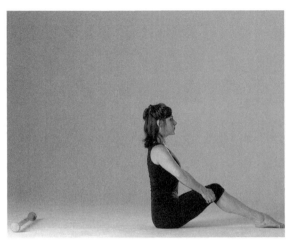

1. Inhale and bend your knees. Sit up tall. Place your hands behind your knees.

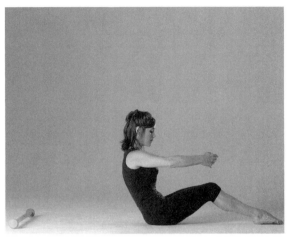

2. Exhale and scoop the abdominals as you round your arms to chest level.

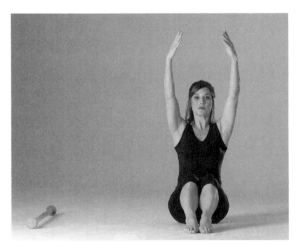

3. Inhale and lengthen your spine as you bring the arms overhead, just in front of your ears.

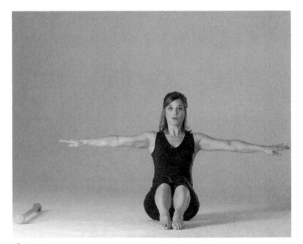

4. Bring your arms to the sides.

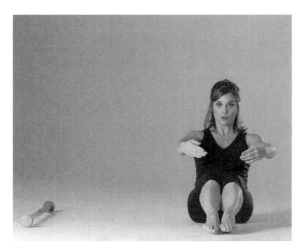

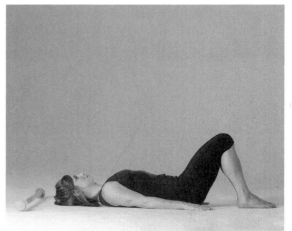

5. Exhale and scoop a little lower as you round your arms to chest level.

6. Repeat this flowing action 4 times.

7. Exhale as you slowly roll down vertebra by vertebra. Slide your feet in and place your arms at your sides to lower completely.

HELPFUL REMINDERS:

- Lengthen your back starting from your tailbone, and continuing up the back to the crown of your head.
- Press your shoulders down as you lift your arms to the sides, overhead, and front.
- Bring your abdominal muscles toward your spine by actively pulling in and up.
- Always inhale to lengthen the spine, and exhale to roll down.

Hips-and-Chest Lift

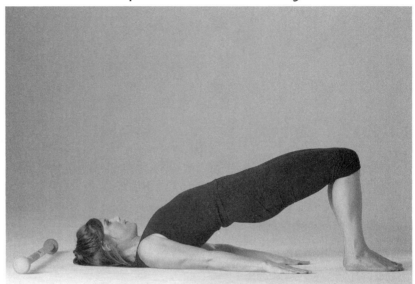

1. Lift your hips and chest up toward the ceiling.

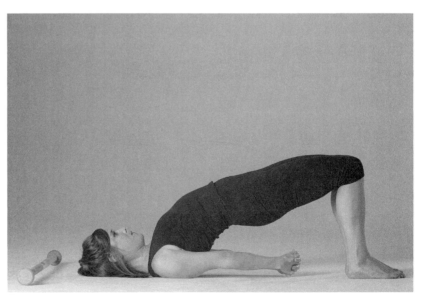

2. Interlace your hands and roll onto the shoulders to stretch and lift higher.

3. Hold this position for 20 seconds.

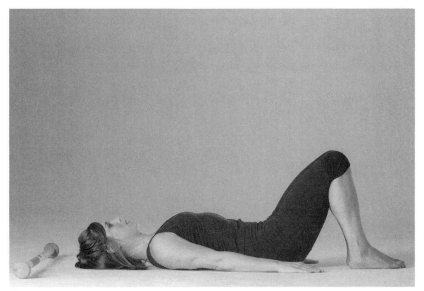

4. Exhale and roll down one vertebra at a time.

The last area to connect to the floor is your tailbone.

5. Lower your trunk completely to the floor.

Align your shoulders, hips, knees, and ankles and lengthen.

H E L P F U L   R E M I N D E R S :

- Firmly press the backs of your arms and hands against the floor.

- Your ankles should be directly underneath your knees.

- Protect your lower back by pulling in the lower abdominals as you lift.

- Close your rib cage.

- Lengthen the fronts of your thighs and hips by reaching them away from your center. Stay completely parallel.

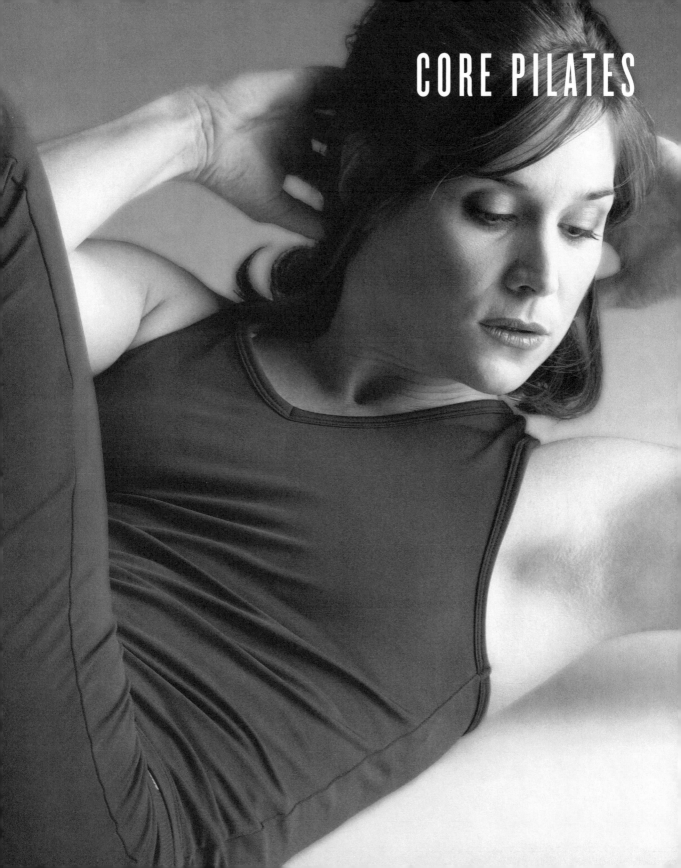

Core Pilates

Developing strong abdominal and lower back muscles will improve your personal workout experience and preclude future problems as you move through life. On a purely practical level, maintaining a strong and healthy core (mainly abs, pelvis, back, and buttocks) protects you from injury and strain in the lower back—a common concern that all of us should be mindful of. Aesthetically, a flat, firm stomach is something to strive for, and is a great accomplishment for those of us who want to see visible rewards from regularly working out. In BalleCore, you quickly target this area and zone in on how to activate your core and stabilize the spine. Remember, the BalleCore philosophy is this: Developing a strong core, and learning to utilize your power from the midsection of your body, will allow you to exercise more efficiently and with greater ease. The core exercises form the basis that will determine how you move through the BalleCore program.

Precision and subtlety are key elements to consider while you are exercising in this section. My cueing will help you learn to recruit your inner muscles rather than overusing your "global" or larger muscles to do the work. Feel free to refer back to the Body Concepts in Getting Started, should you need a quick refresher course.

Benefits:

- ❏ Strengthens your inner muscles and prepares the body to work as a whole.
- ❏ Develops strong abdominal muscles—transverse, oblique, and rectus.
- ❏ Protects the back from injury.
- ❏ Builds endurance and confidence with movement.

Core Curl-Ups

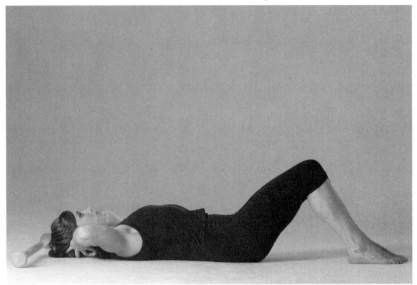

1. Place your hands behind your head and inhale.

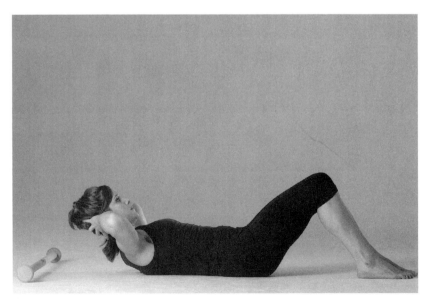

2. Exhale as you peel your head, neck, and upper shoulders off the floor.

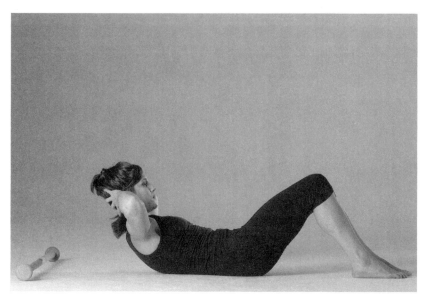

3. Continue to exhale as you focus your eyes at the top of your knees, creating a scooped position.

4. Inhale at the same time that you lower onto the floor.

REPEAT 8 TIMES

Core Curl-Ups with Pulse

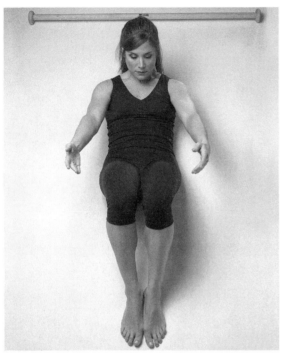

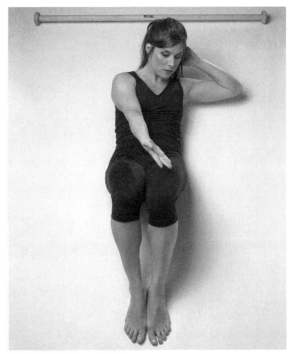

1. Exhale, and lift to your Core Curl-Up position. Release your arms and stretch them in line with your knees. Gently pulse your arms as you breathe in and out for 8 pulses.

2. Rotate your upper trunk so your right arm is reaching toward the left knee, and pulse 8 times. Your left hand is behind your head, with the elbow touching the floor.

HELPFUL REMINDERS:

- Press your lower back into the floor, or imprint, without tucking your pelvis.
- Engage your buttock muscles and inner thighs without overusing, by gripping.
- Keep your knees in line, with your hip bones pointing up to the ceiling.
- Focus on full exhalations to facilitate deep contractions within your core muscles, specifically your obliques.
- Soften your breastbone and neck as you lift your head off the floor.
- Anytime your head is lifted, the base of your shoulder blades should be touching the mat. This ensures proper positioning and will relieve tension.
- Draw your shoulder blades down the back, creating a V. Your upper back is broadened as your lower back feels more compact.
- Keep your elbow on the mat as you cross over.
- The soles of your feet should be firmly on the floor and in parallel.

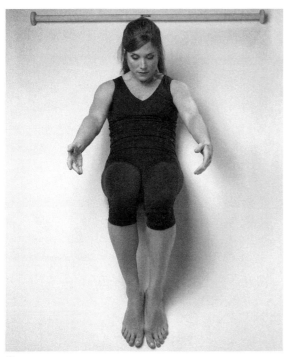 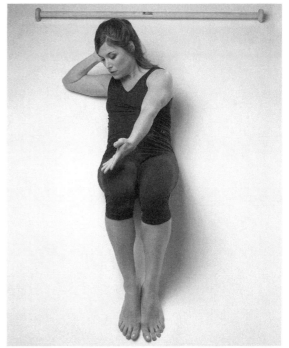

3. Come back to the center, and reach and pulse both arms toward the knees 8 times.

4. Switch to the other side, release your left arm, and pulse toward the right knee for 8 pulses. Your right hand is behind your head, with the elbow touching the floor.

5. Repeat the crossover pulses 2 times.

6. Place your hands behind your head and inhale to lower.

Butterfly Curl-Ups with Port de Bras

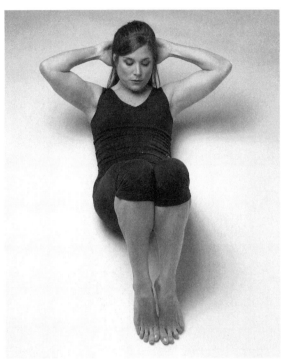

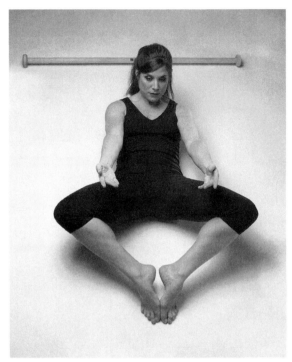

1. Inhale, with your hands behind your head and the soles of your feet on the floor. Exhale as you curl up and slide your feet closer to your body. Press your lower back into the floor.

2. Open your knees symmetrically and pulse your arms, breathing in and out for 8 pulses.

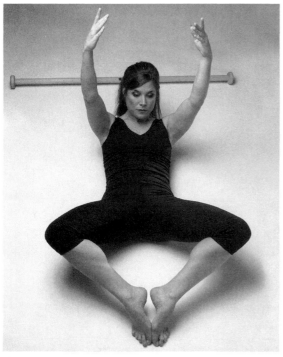

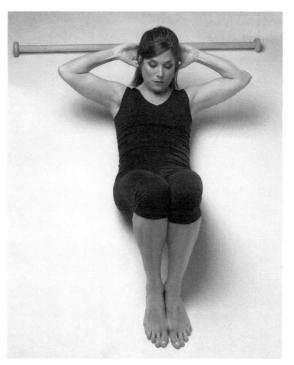

3. Inhale and bring your arms to your ears to fifth port de bras, without changing your body position.

4. Place your hands behind your head and squeeze your inner thighs together. Roll down to finish.

REPEAT 3 TIMES

HELPFUL REMINDERS:

- By bringing your ribs closer to the hips as you pulse you enable the abdominal muscles to contract.
- Connect your abdominals to the lower back.
- Your arms are firm, not stiff. Your elbows and wrists are slightly rounded.
- Broaden your chest as you reach your arms forward and overhead.

Core Breathing with Port de Bras

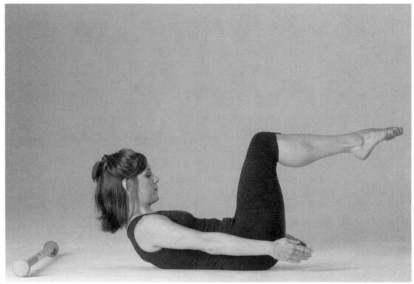

1. Bring your head up to your Core Curl-Up position and bend your knees in line with your hip bones. Your legs are at a right angle, and your arms are slightly rounded at the hips.

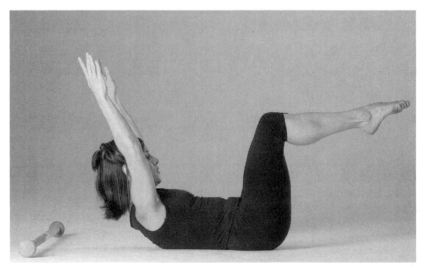

2. Inhale, and bring your arms overhead to fifth port de bras.

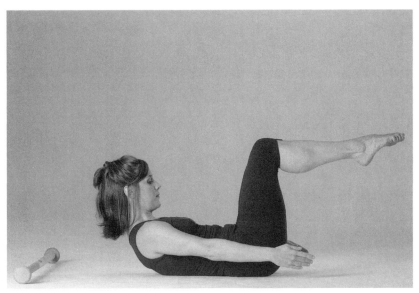

3. Fully exhale as you sweep the arms out to the sides and back to your hips.

4. Repeat steps 2 and 3 eight times.

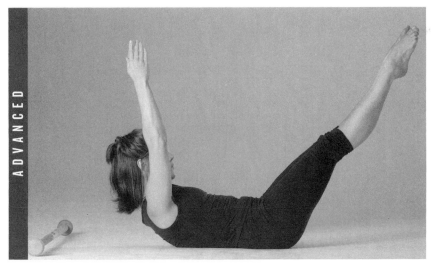

ADVANCED

5. Extend your legs out to your point of control (somewhere between a 45- and 60-degree angle).

6. Continue with steps 2 and 3 eight more times.

7. Bend the knees and lower your head. Repeat 8 times.

REPEAT 2 TIMES

Half Roll-Up (Transitional Move)

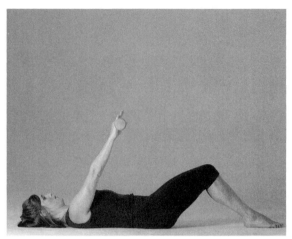

1. Inhale, stretch your arms overhead, and reach for your stretch band or BalleCore Barre.

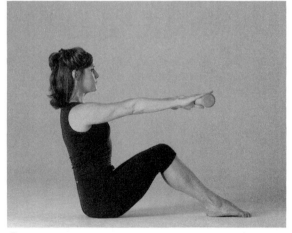

2. Exhale completely as you bring your barre up to chest level. Knit the ribs together. Now begin to peel off the floor, starting at your neck.

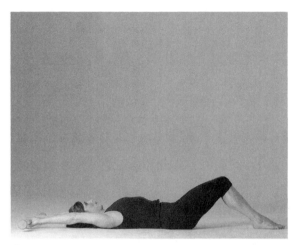

3. Slowly inhale as you continue to peel your body off the floor, scooping out your abdominals.

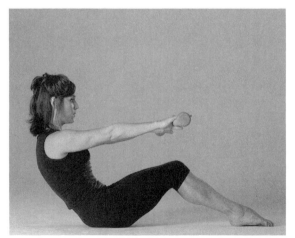

4. Exhale, and sit up tall, lengthening your trunk and lifting out of your waist.

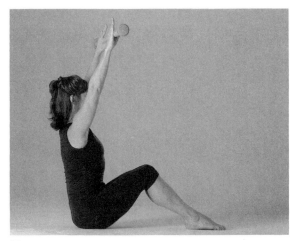

5. Inhale, and reach your barre overhead.

6. Exhale, press your barre back to chest level, and roll down with control.

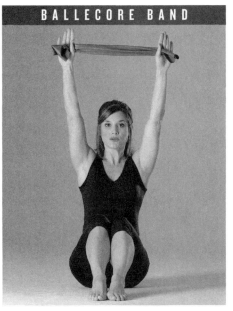

BALLECORE BAND

Use your BalleCore Barre or Band as a resistance tool and guide for proper alignment in your body.

REPEAT 2 TIMES

HELPFUL REMINDERS:

- Keep your breathing fluid and connected to the movement.
- Your rib cage must be closed and your belly must be pulled into the floor to initiate the roll-up.
- Focus on symmetry in your body. Keep your shoulders square, hips in line, and inner thighs activated.

CORE PILATES VARIATION: *Pedaling*

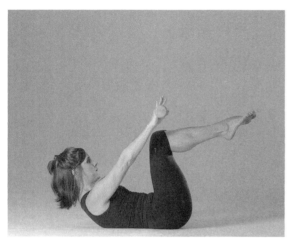

1. Lift your head and bring your knees and ankles in line with your hips.

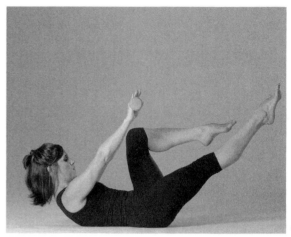

2. Push through the base of your toes and balls of the feet as you alternate drawing your knee into your chest while the opposite leg reaches away.

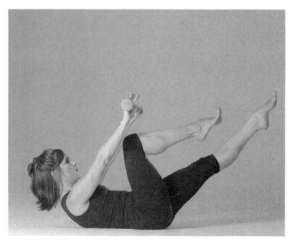

3. Bring both knees in and lower your head if needed, or continue to the next exercise.

REPEAT 6 TIMES

CORE PILATES VARIATION: *Push-Through*

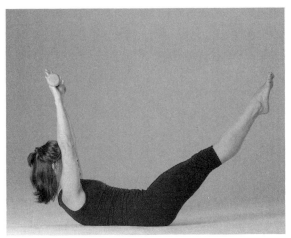

1. Inhale and extend your arms and legs simultaneously as you remain anchored in the center.

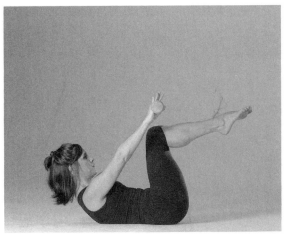

2. Exhale and draw your arms and legs into your body.

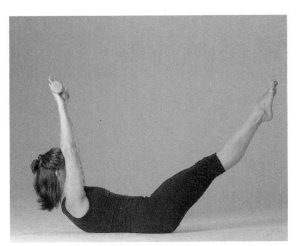

3. Inhale and reach your arms and push your legs out simultaneously as you stay anchored in your center.

REPEAT 6 TIMES

CORE PILATES VARIATION: *Leg Splits*

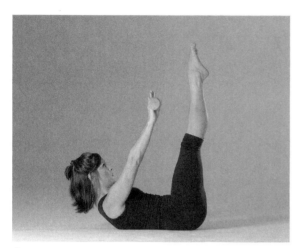

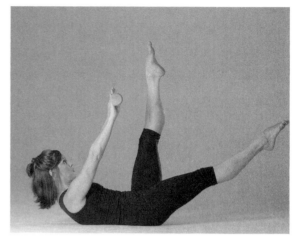

1. Keep your head up and bring your legs to the ceiling. Continue to focus on your breathing.

2. Inhale and lower your right leg halfway down. Exhale and bring your leg back up to 90 degrees.

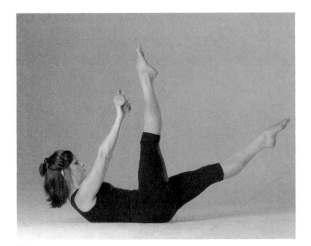

3. Alternate with your left leg.

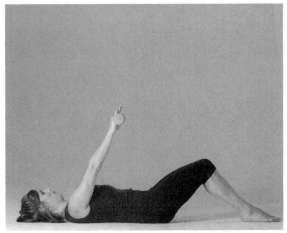

4. Lower your head and legs to the floor.

REPEAT 3 TIMES

HELPFUL REMINDERS:

- Lower your head and rest between exercises if you are feeling strain.
- Your inner thigh and buttock muscles must be working along with your abdominals.
- The BalleCore Barre never reaches beyond your ears while your head is lifted.
- As you draw the knees into the body, pull your abdominal muscles deeper into your center.
- If your back arches, this is an indication that you are lowering your legs too far.
- The tailbone should never come off the floor.
- Stay focused.

Half Can-Can

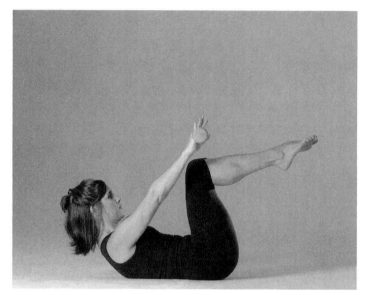

1. Bring your knees and head into your Core Curl-Up
position and inhale.

HELPFUL REMINDERS:

- Keep your knees and inner thighs seamed together as you slightly shift from side to side.
  Your elbows do not need to touch your knees.

- Your eyes should follow the arms.

- Keep pulling your waist in as you exhale.

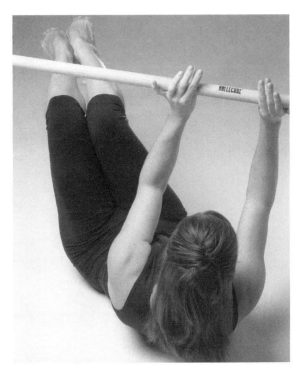

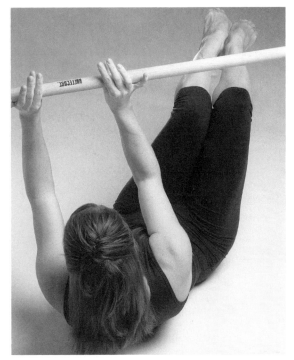

2. Slide your arms in so they are about 6 inches apart and in line with the inside of your shoulders. Bend your elbows to form a right angle.

3. Exhale, slightly rotate your trunk, and aim your right elbow toward the opposite (left) hip bone. Keeping your knees together, shift your legs slightly to the right to counterbalance your body. Alternate 6 times side to side by passing through and pressing your lower back into the floor.

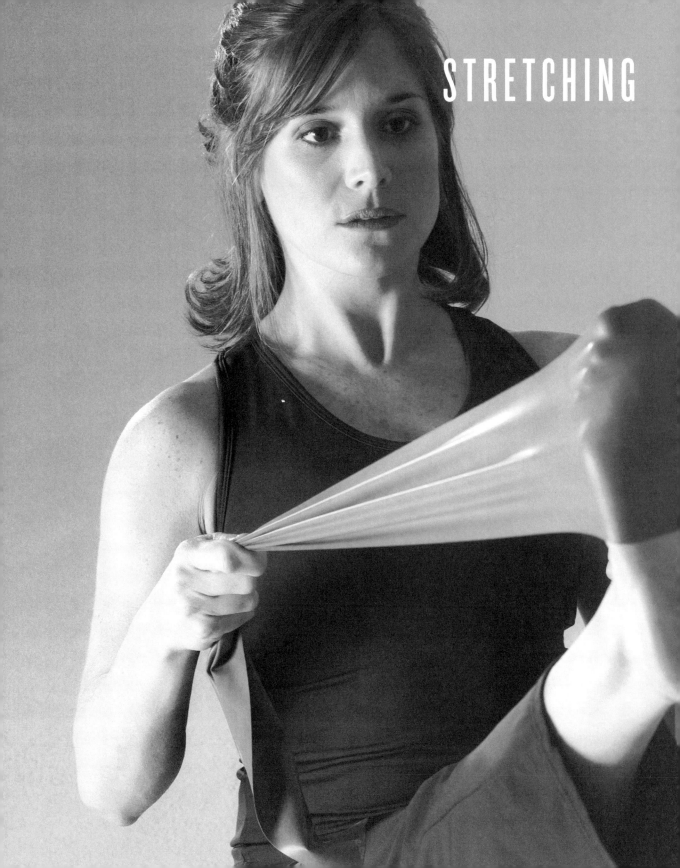

STRETCHING

Stretching

In life's journey, we all are susceptible to accumulating tension, from both emotional tribulations and physical pain. Stretching regularly can ease this burden and make positive changes in your body. I have chosen wonderful, effective stretches that target common tight areas such as the hips, hamstrings, and back. These areas are where you habitually hold tension and are often the cause of physical aches and pains. Such pains accumulate whether you lead a sedentary lifestyle or play competitive sports. Increasing mobility in the hip area permits blood to circulate more freely between the legs and torso.

The following exercises target the hips and bottom, creating better muscle tone and more mobility. Your structural base is made up of your hips, gluteals, and lumbar spine, which support your inner core. The hip area affects simple and complex movement patterns. If you experience lower back pain or even shoulder pain, you may be suffering from the effects of inflexible hip muscles. Stiffness in the hip joint can have adverse effects on the spine, knees, and feet. This tightness can pull you forward and misalign the entire body. You can benefit from properly strengthening and stretching the muscles that attach the hips to your pelvis by experimenting with these stretches.

Stretching is essential within the BalleCore program, and I recommend doing these exercises daily to keep your body balanced and healthy. The result is increased flexibility plus longer-looking leg muscles. At the same time, you benefit from your mind shifting into a more relaxed and focused state, which adds confidence to your movements.

Your posture is also affected by imbalances in the body. Too much strength in any area of the body can indicate tightness, and too much flexibility can represent a weakness. Muscular symmetry—striking a balance between stretching the muscles and strengthening them—is requisite for supporting your structural foundation. Stretching not only feels amazing but, done regularly, also infuses you with renewed energy and vitality.

Benefits:

- ❑ Releases the inner thighs (adductors), outer thighs (abductors), hip flexors, back, and feet.
- ❑ Promotes youthfulness and flexibility in the spine.
- ❑ Creates equilibrium in the body.
- ❑ Reduces fatigue and stiffness in the body.

STRETCHING VARIATION: *Hamstring Stretch*

Remember: Perform all lying down or supine exercises with the same leg before switching to the other side. The stretches flow from one to the next to open up tight muscles and joints.

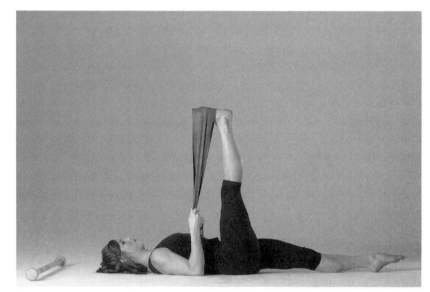

1. Place the stretch band wide over your right foot. Hold on to each end of the band with your elbows at your sides. Hold the stretch for 30 seconds.

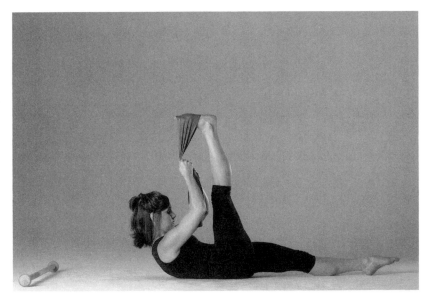

2. Lift your head, neck, upper back, and elbows off the floor, and stretch your hamstring further by gently bringing your head closer to your leg.

3. Roll down slowly and lengthen your body on the mat.

4. Breathe naturally.

STRETCHING VARIATION: *Inner Thigh and Hip Stretch*

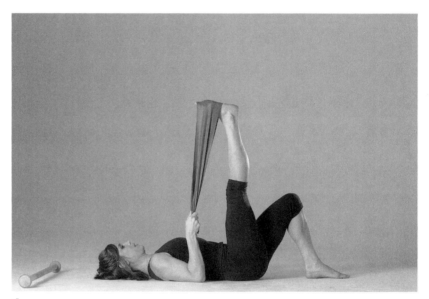

1. Slide your left foot in so that your knee is facing up. Hold the band with your right hand.

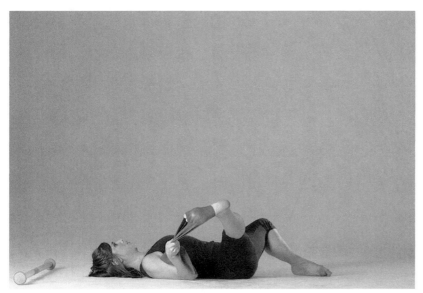

2. Inhale and place your left hand on your left hip. Slowly open the legs simultaneously.

3. Exhale, bringing both of your legs up to starting position to face up.

REPEAT 4 TIMES

STRETCHING VARIATION: *Grand Leg Circles*

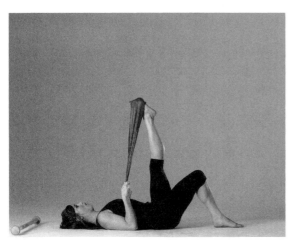 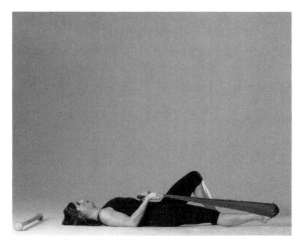

1. Hold on to each end of the band with your elbows at your sides. Push through the ball of the foot to lengthen your leg muscles.

2. Lower your right leg as you reach out of your hips, down toward the floor.

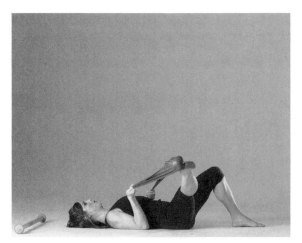

3. Carry your leg out to the side.

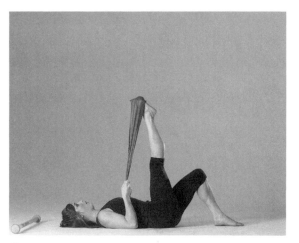

4. Bring your leg back up to the ceiling. Reverse directions.

REPEAT 4 TIMES

ADVANCED

1. Fully extend your left leg, keeping it firm against the floor as you circle the right leg.

STRETCHING VARIATION: *Point-and-Flex Walk-Up*

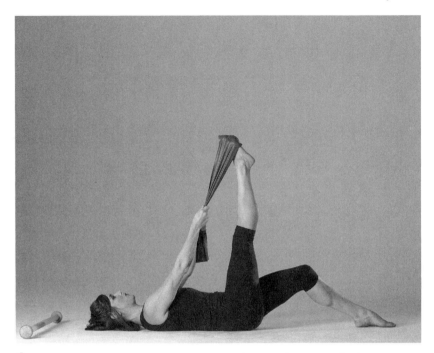

1. Inhale, and bend your left knee and extend your right leg to the ceiling. Hold on firmly with your band.

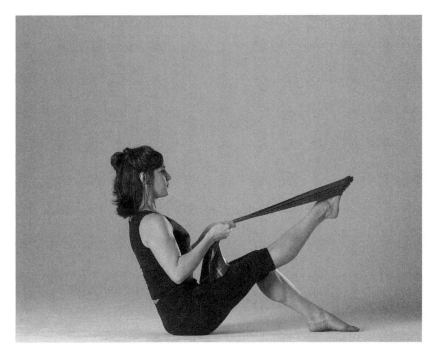

2. Exhale and roll off the floor to walk up your leg, engaging your abdominals. Point and flex the foot several times.

HELPFUL REMINDERS:

- Create length from the top of your head to your toes.
- Align your shoulders, hips, knees, and ankles.
- Maintain control within your body, yet allow your muscles to release.
- Continue to breathe rhythmically as you stretch the muscles and progress to the next exercise, creating continuity.
- You can create more, or less, resistance with the band by changing your grip and hand placement.

STRETCHING VARIATION: *Torso Twist*

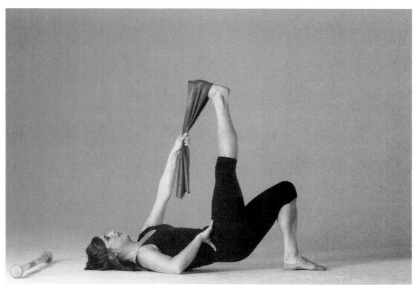

1. With your left foot, lift your left side off the mat for a moment, and shift your left hip to the center of the mat.

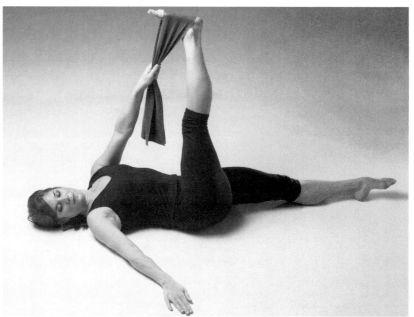

2. Exhale, and straighten both legs. Slowly cross your right leg over to your left.

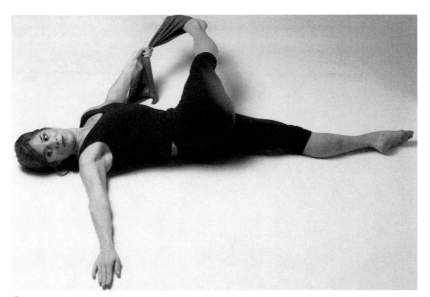

3. Continue to rotate your torso and leg to the left. Feel your upper back opening up and your midback releasing. Hold the stretch, breathing in and out.

4. Inhale and draw your abdominal muscles into your back and side muscles. Carefully bring your leg back up to the ceiling as you roll your back onto the floor. Reach for your band with both hands.

SEATED: *Point-and-Flex*

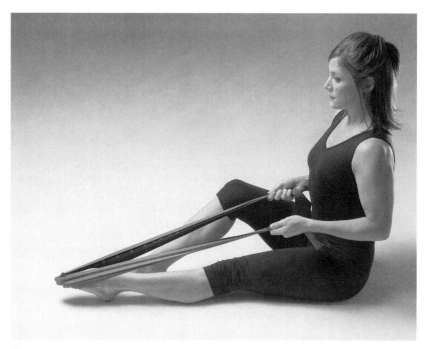

1. Sit upright, keeping your elbows at your sides. Bend your right knee and extend your left leg. Point your foot.

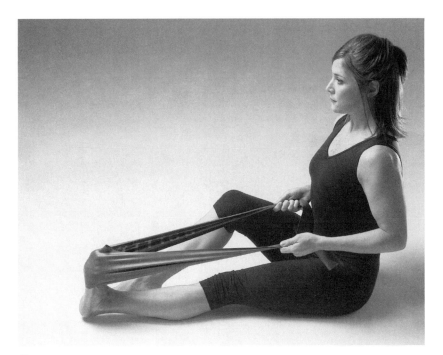

2. Flex your foot.

3. Continue pointing and flexing your foot 8 times.

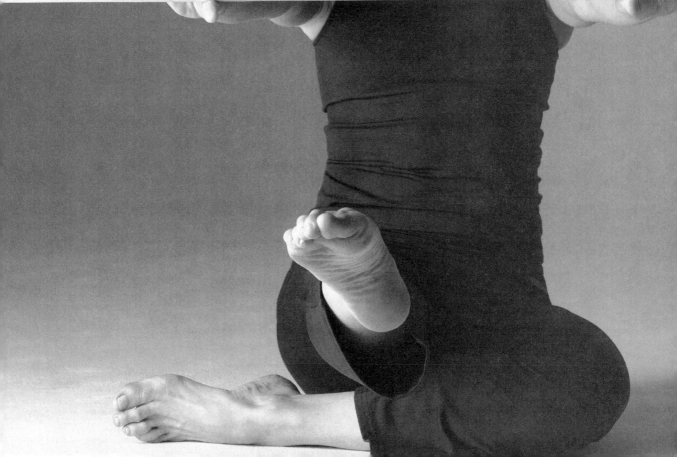

Hips and Buttocks

If you look at children playing, notice the freedom and boundless energy that their physicality allows them. The regular lives of healthy children take them through countless movements, twisting, turning, and tumbling from one direction swiftly into the next. If you think about the directions your own body revolves in, you may come up with only a couple: front and back. Moving in a circular motion in an exercise class is not the norm. In BalleCore, we take things several steps farther by reeducating the muscles and joints to move in different movement patterns, focusing on rotation. The hips are capable of a wide range of motion in more than two directions, and the rewards of creating muscle equilibrium are endless. You'll open the back and free the hips by expanding your range of motion using circular movements throughout the workout.

Benefits:

❏ Shapes the hips, buttocks, and thighs.
❏ Creates fluidity in the back.
❏ Trims inches from the waist.

Full Roll-Up (Transitional Move)

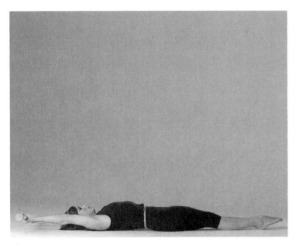

1. Stretch your body long with your arms at your sides and your legs pulled together tightly. Inhale and stretch your arms overhead. Reach for your BalleCore Barre or Band.

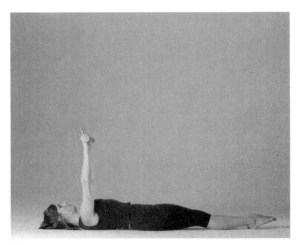

2. Exhale and bring your barre up to the ceiling as you knit your ribs together and engage your abdominals. Slide your shoulders down.

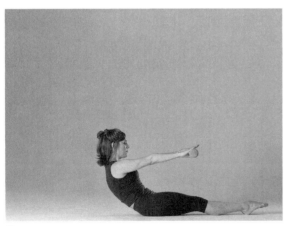

3. Peel off your mat vertebra by vertebra, remaining scooped.

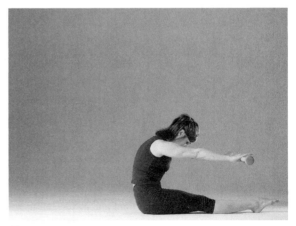

4. Continue to stretch your arms forward at shoulder level and scoop your abdominals. Let your head relax forward.

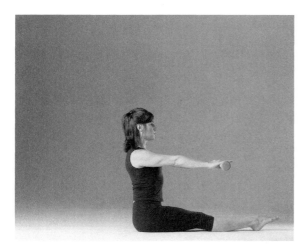

5. Roll through your spine, starting from your lower back and continuing up your spine, then sit up tall.

If you are having difficulty rolling off the mat, try bending your knees and follow steps 1 through 4.

HELPFUL REMINDERS:

- Keep your breathing fluid and connected to the movement.
- Your rib cage must be closed and your belly must be pulled into the floor to initiate the roll-up.
- Focus on symmetry in the body. Keep your shoulders square, hips in line, and inner thighs activated.
- Use your BalleCore Barre or Band as a resistance tool and guide for alignment.
- Transitional moves from one to the next are just as important as any other, making your exercise experience fluid.

UPPER BACK VARIATION: *Forward Roll*

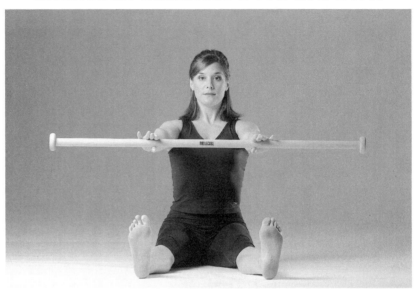

1. Open your legs about 2 to 3 inches outside your shoulders.
Your arms should be in line with your chest. Push through your
heels and balls of your feet to activate your legs. Lift off your seat
and lengthen the torso; inhale.

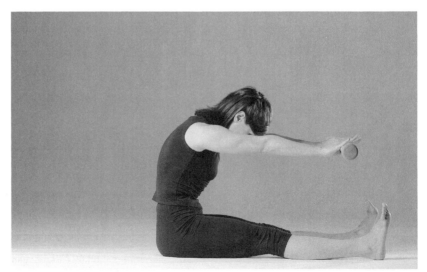

2. Exhale and scoop your stomach. Allow your head, neck,
shoulders, and upper back to stretch forward. Your arms
stay at chest level.

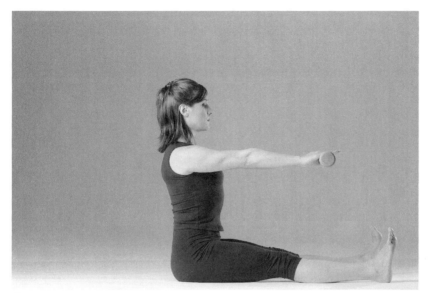

3. Roll back up through your spine one vertebra at a time, starting from your midback and continuing to the top of your head.

REPEAT 3 TIMES

HELPFUL REMINDERS:

- Push through your heels and activate your thighs.
- Roll your shoulders back and lift your sternum.
- Draw your abdominals in and up. Knit your ribs.
- Lengthen from the top of your head.
- Anchor your sitting bones into the floor.

UPPER BACK VARIATION: *Cambré to the Side*

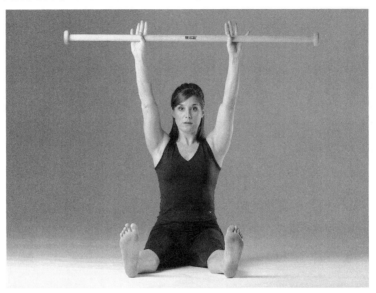

1. Inhale and reach your barre overhead.

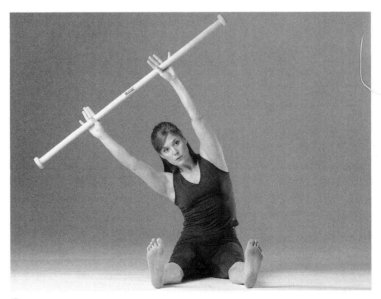

2. Exhale, and slightly bend your torso to the right, or cambré to the side, stacking your ribs.

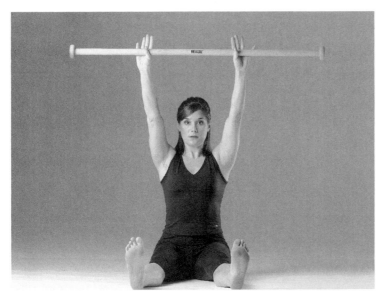

3. Inhale, and lift your barre overhead.

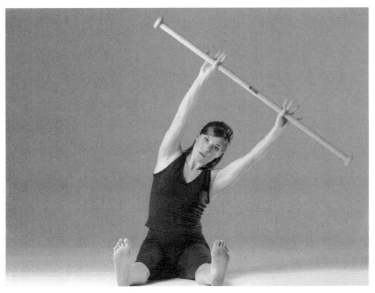

4. Exhale, and slightly bend your torso to your left,
or cambré to the side, stacking your ribs.

R E P E A T   3   T I M E S

UPPER BACK VARIATION: *Semicircle*

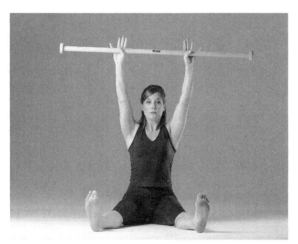

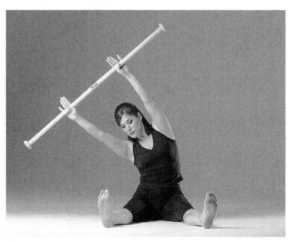

1. Inhale, and reach your barre overhead, slightly in front of your ears.

2. Exhale, and bend your torso to your right, or cambré to the side, stacking your ribs.

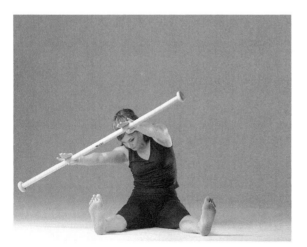

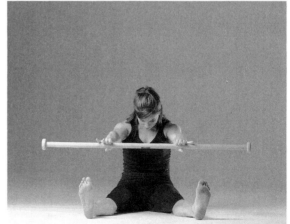

3. Keeping the barre at chest level, continue rounding your upper torso forward, passing through your center, or cambré en rond.

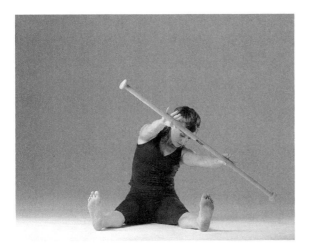

4. Move your arms and upper torso to your left side.

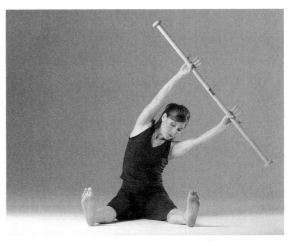

5. Exhale, and slightly bend your torso to your left, stacking your ribs.

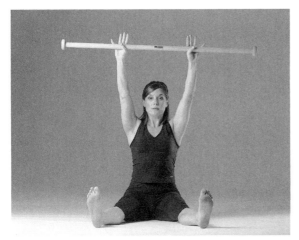

6. Inhale, and reach your barre overhead. Repeat in both directions.

HELPFUL REMINDERS:

- Anchor your lower body by energizing your legs.
- Gently squeeze your buttock muscles and pull your belly inward toward the back.
- Lengthen your torso, reaching out of your waist, keeping your hips quiet.
- While bending your torso from side to side, stay lifted. Reach up before stretching sideways.
- Keep these movements fluid and circular, and exhale completely.
- Roll your shoulder blades back to broaden your chest and improve your posture.

REPEAT 3 TIMES

SEATED FAN VARIATION: *Rolls*

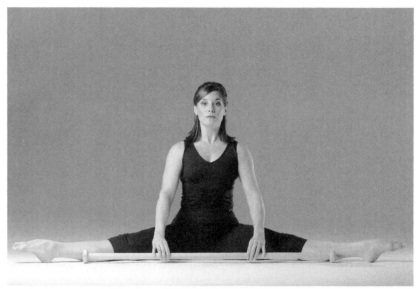

1. Open your legs wide and stretch your feet. Starting at the base of your spine, slowly straighten your back and inhale.

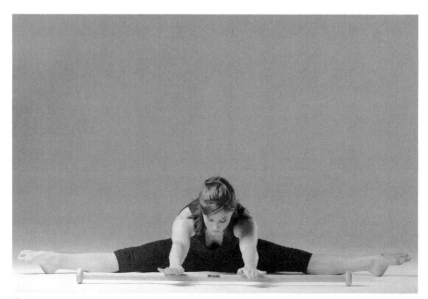

2. With or without your barre, slowly stretch your upper body forward toward the floor. Keep your legs activated, with your knees facing up to the ceiling, and exhale.

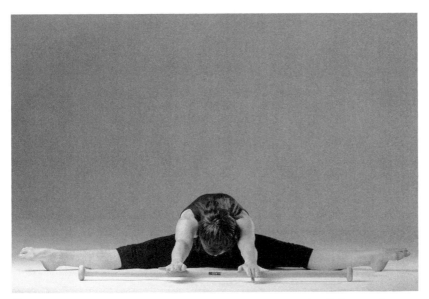

3. Allow your entire spine and neck to stretch and roll forward. Breathe in and out several times.

4. Press firmly on your barre, keeping your shoulders in place as you roll up one vertebra at a time. Inhale.

REPEAT 3 TIMES

SEATED FAN VARIATION: *Diagonal Reaches*

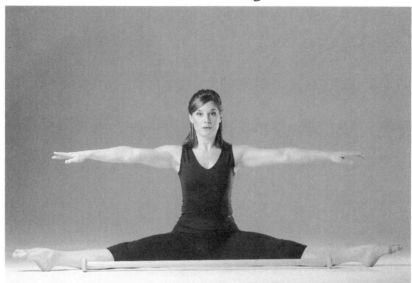

1. Extend both arms to your sides at chest level.

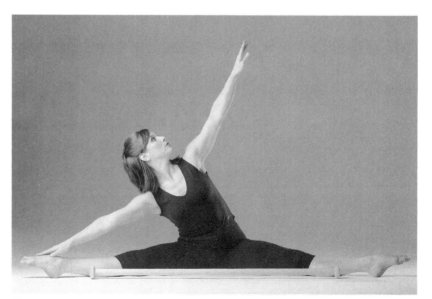

2. Stretch and reach your right arm to your right ankle while at the same time extending your left arm to the diagonal, creating a long line. Look to your left arm.

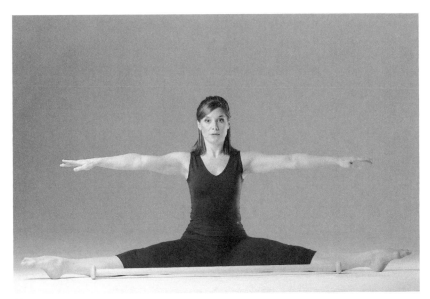

3. Extend both arms to your sides.

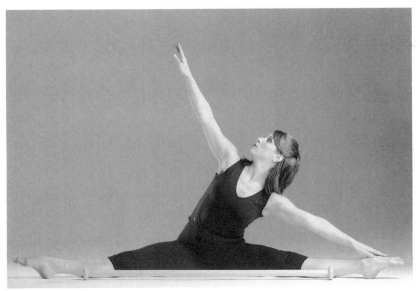

4. Stretch and reach your left arm to your left ankle while at the same time extending your right arm to the diagonal, creating a long line. Look to your right arm.

5. Extend both arms back to your sides.

REPEAT 3 TIMES

SEATED FAN VARIATION: *Around the World*

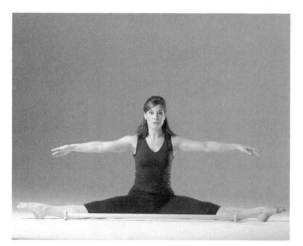

1. Extend your arms out to your sides, or to second port de bras.

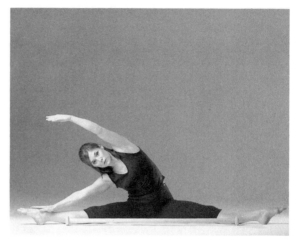

2. Bring your left arm overhead and stretch over to your right leg.

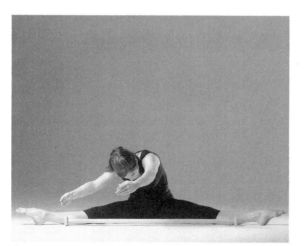

3. Round your back forward toward the center of your body, with both arms overhead.

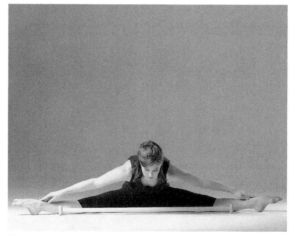

4. As your torso passes directly through your center, reach your left arm to meet your left leg. Release your right arm and round your body over to your left side.

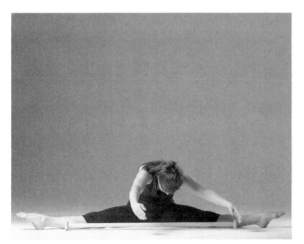

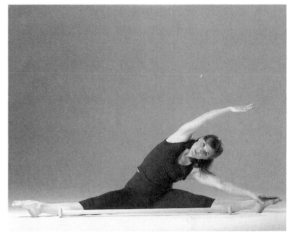

5. Stretch your right arm overhead and reach sideways to your left.

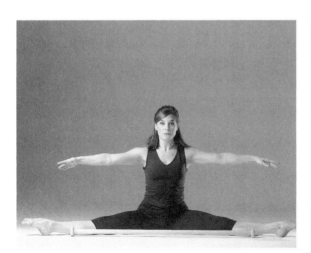

6. Stretch up and bring your arms out to your sides. Repeat the exercise.

7. Repeat 3 times in both directions.

HELPFUL REMINDERS:

- Around the World creates mobility in your torso through circular motion.

- Keep your kneecaps facing up toward the ceiling throughout the Seated Fan variation.

- Avoid tilting your pelvis forward or back. If your hamstrings are tight or your back is not erect, bend your knees.

- Your thighs should stay firm against the floor, and your toes should stay pointed.

- Your arms should be stretched and never locked at the elbows.

- While you are stretching sideways, the sides of your ribs should be parallel to your thighs to feel the maximum stretch.

- When your arms are extended to your sides, your fingers should be in your peripheral vision.

PRETZEL POSITION VARIATION: *Hip Lifts*

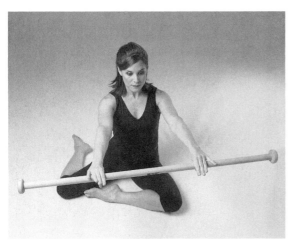

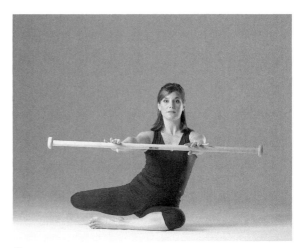

1. Bring your left knee and foot into the front of your body and bend your right knee so that it is in line with your right hip bone. This is your pretzel position. The BalleCore Barre should be at chest level.

2. Lift your back (right) leg off the floor. Lift and lower 8 times.

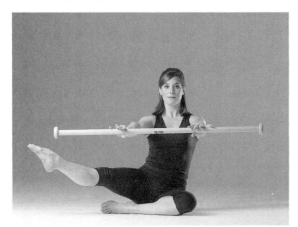

3. Fully extend your right leg to the side, with the knee facing up.

and Rond de Jambes with BalleCore Barre

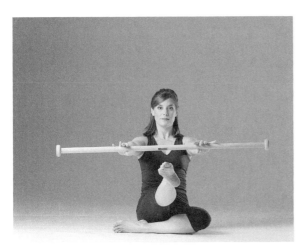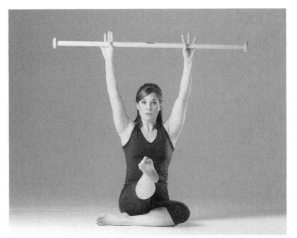

4. Reach out of your hip and continue wrapping the leg to the front of your body, leading with your heel. Your kneecap should be facing away. This action is a rond de jambe.

5. Inhale, raise your barre up overhead, and exhale to bring it back to chest level.

6. Leading with the pointed foot, wrap the leg around to the back, keeping the leg fully extended until it passes at the hip. Bend your knee to the back, stretching your thigh away and contracting your buttocks.

7. Repeat steps 3 through 6 six times.

8. Lower the right leg.

9. Repeat the sequence with the left leg behind.

PRETZEL POSITION VARIATION: *Hip Lifts*

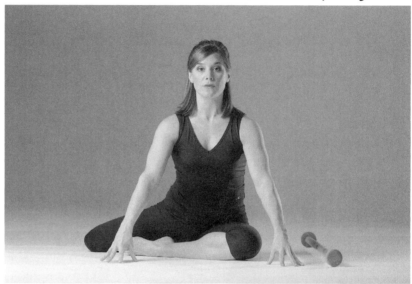

1. Follow steps 1 through 9, but firmly place your fingertips in front of your body to keep you lifted. When your arms are at your sides, reach your fingers long. When the arms go to the back, firmly place your fingertips behind you to keep you lifted.

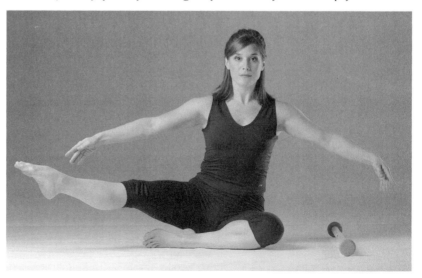

and Rond de Jambes without BalleCore Barre

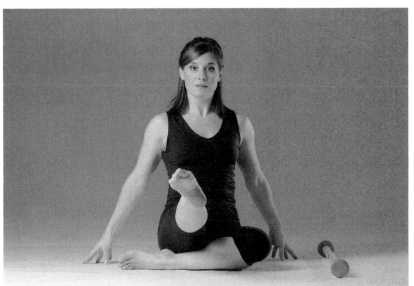

HELPFUL REMINDERS:

- Lower or change the position of the barre at any time to make the exercise more comfortable or challenging for you.

- Pulling up and using your core muscles will help you lift the working leg.

- Breathe rhythmically in and out.

- Square off your shoulders and hips to begin. Keep your torso lifted throughout.

- Try not to swing your leg or let your leg drop as you lift and lower. Maintain control and move at a steady pace.

- Reach your working leg out of the hips to lengthen your muscles.

- Keep your working leg on the same plane as it moves from front to back.

- Lower onto your forearm if the Pretzel Position is difficult. In time, the hips will release.

Hip and Thigh Press

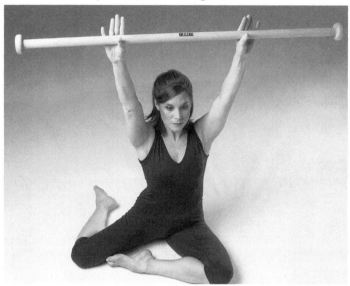

1. In your Pretzel Position, inhale deeply and bring your arms overhead.

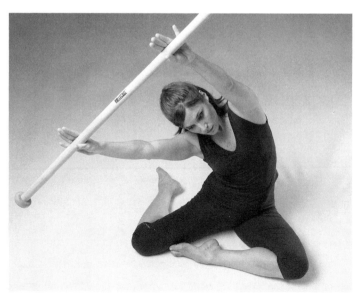

2. Fully exhale and bend or cambré to the side.

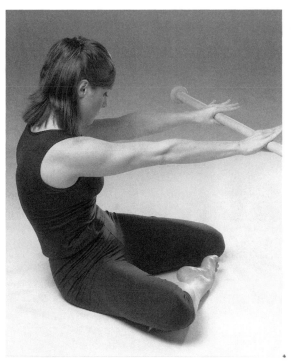

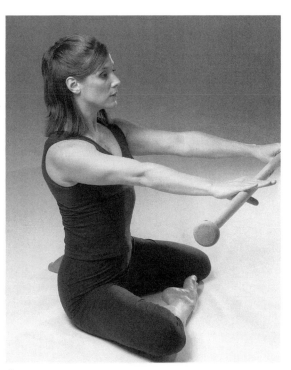

3. Simultaneously, round the barre to the front of your body then again to chest level, and contract the abdominal muscles as you scoop deeply into your lower back. Press your inner thighs into the floor. Hold for five seconds.

4. Straighten your back to finish.

REPEAT 3 TIMES

HELPFUL REMINDERS:

- Lengthen from your waist up to completely stretch the back.
- Feel the resistance as you reach the barre away, at the same time pulling your abdominals into your back.
- Firmly press your inner thigh, groin, and hip area into the floor to enhance the stretch and muscle release.

TORSO AND HIP TWIST VARIATION: *To the Side*

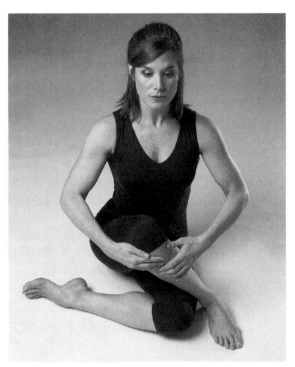

1. Cross your right leg over the left. The sole of your right foot should be on the floor. Gently pull your right knee into your chest and extend your torso, starting from the base of your spine.

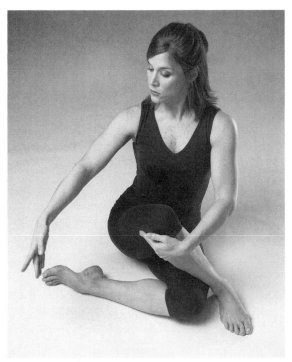 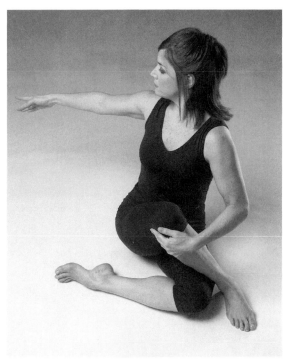

2. Inhale, then lift and twist your trunk as you reach your right arm to the back.

3. Exhale, and bring your right arm back to starting position.

4. Repeat with your left arm. Continue with the next exercise.

REPEAT 2 TIMES

TORSO AND HIP TWIST VARIATION: *To the Center*

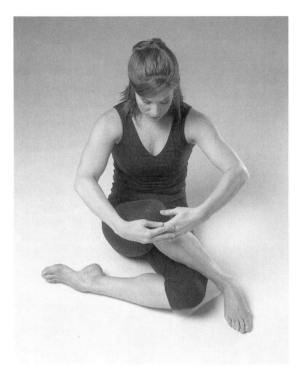 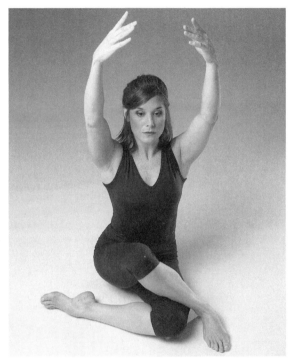

1. In the same position, exhale, and contract your abdominal muscles by scooping into the lower back. Grasp the outside of the knees and hold the stretch.

2. Inhale then and extend your torso and draw the arms up overhead to fifth port de bras position.

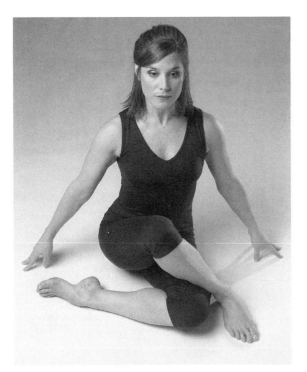

3. Continue to exhale and reach your arms to your sides. Lift and open your chest, and stretch your arms and fingertips just behind the hips. Switch leg positions or go to the next exercise.

REPEAT 2 TIMES

TORSO AND HIP TWIST VARIATION: *To the Floor*
(ADVANCED STRETCH)

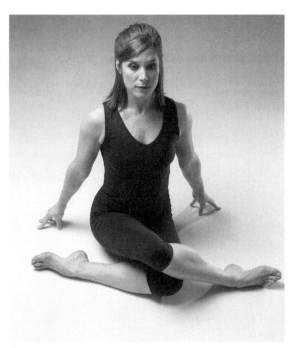

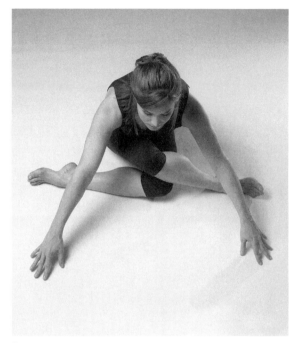

1. Lift your chest and stretch the arms and fingertips just behind your hips. Allow your right leg to relax over the left. Your knees should be stacked, your shins are relaxed as you gently push your ankles away from your body.

2. Walk your fingertips to the front. Bending from your hips, stretch your arms and torso to the floor for a deeper stretch within your hip area. Exhale.

3. Hold the stretch for 15 seconds.

4. Walk your hands and torso back as you roll up.

5. Inhale, and straighten your back completely. Perform the Torso and Hips Twist Variation with the left leg on top.

H E L P F U L   R E M I N D E R S :

- To release tension in your hip area, it's important to breathe rhythmically in and out.

- Engage your buttock muscles to avoid falling back off your sitting bones.

- As you twist sideways, allow your eyes to follow your hand.

- Bring your knee into your chest as close as possible to increase the stretch in your lower back, hips, and thighs.

- Always keep the chest up and shoulders back.

- The To the Floor exercise should not be attempted if you have knee problems.

SIDE-LYING VARIATION: *Coupé–Passé–Sous-Sus*

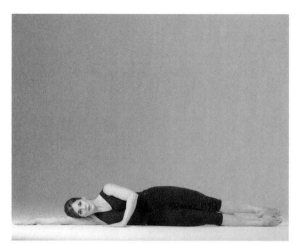

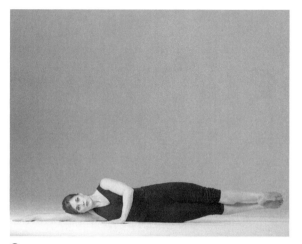

1. Lie on your right side in one straight line. Align your ankles, knees, hips, ribs, and shoulders. Rest your head on your right arm and firmly place your left hand in front of your body to help support you.

2. Cross your left leg over your right leg so that your left ankle is in front of the right one. This is sous-sus. Inhale and lift your bottom (right) leg off the floor. Both legs should be pulled together tightly.

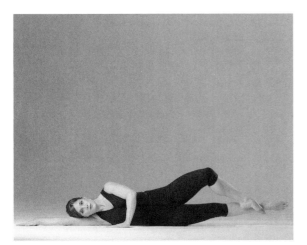

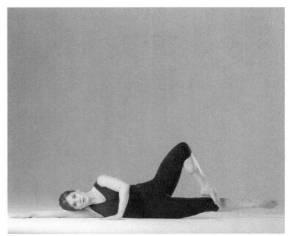

3. Point your left foot and slowly draw your foot up the leg, starting at your ankle, or coupé. The foot should be touching your opposite leg.

4. Continue to slide your left foot up your right leg until it reaches your knee, or passé. Your left leg should be turned out and open, as your knee points directly up to the ceiling.

5. Keep your right leg off the floor and slowly slide your left leg down the front of your leg.

6. Continue to lift your right leg off the floor. The legs should be crossed at your ankles. Hold this position for five seconds.

7. Release your right leg and align your left leg on top.

REPEAT 3 TIMES

SIDE-LYING VARIATION: *Side-Lying Piqué*

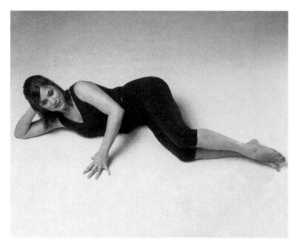

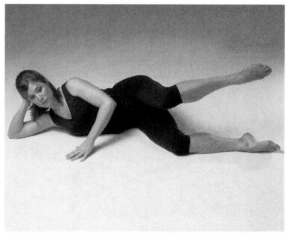

1. Shift your legs forward, making a 45-degree angle. Rest your head in the palm of your hand. Stack your knees and inner thighs, keeping your ankles in line with your knees.

2. Lift the top leg, keeping your hips stacked and facing front.

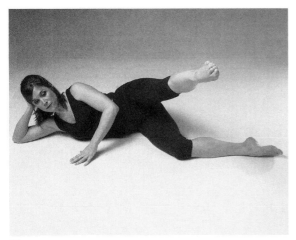

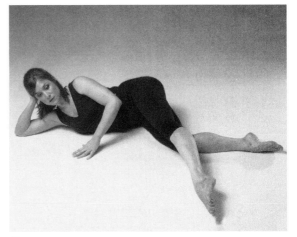

3. Extend your top leg with your toes pointed.

4. Quickly, but with control, lower your leg to the floor and tap your foot to the floor. Bring your straightened leg back up. Keep your leg at the same angle as your hips. Repeat this action 8 times.

5. Bend your knee and close. Repeat the Side-Lying Variation on your left side.

HELPFUL REMINDERS:

- While performing the side-lying exercises, using your core muscles will help you build endurance and perform the movements with more control.
- Engage your abdominal muscles even further by actively lifting your waist off the floor.
- Pull your rib cage in and bring your shoulders back.
- Release tension in your neck by gently resting your head in your hands and keeping your neck long.

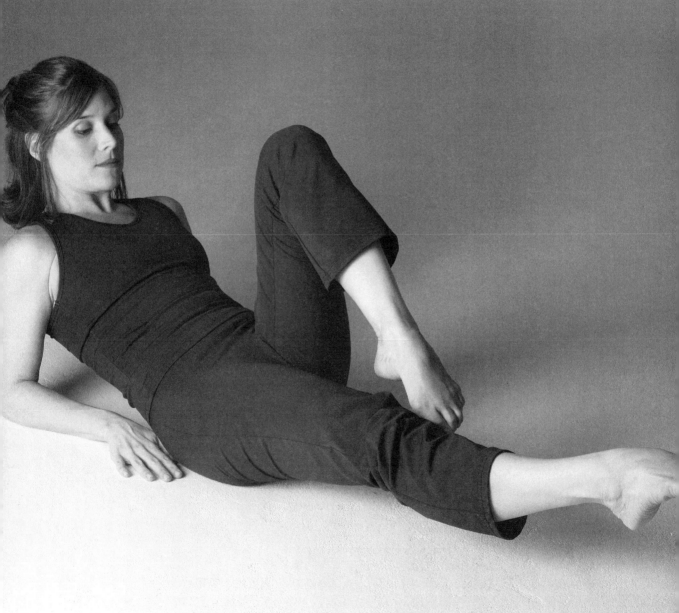

Floor Ballet

These targeted exercises are designed to challenge you by introducing traditional yet dynamic ballet moves on the floor while paying close attention to proper placement and articulation throughout the joints and limbs. The focus is on creating long and elegant lines in the body. Combined with more difficult core-strengthening exercises, these movements will help you improve full body control and endurance. For the most part, this section is easy to follow, but some exercises may not be simple the first time around, so follow the instructions at your own pace.

Benefits:

❑ Sharpens the mind.
❑ Builds endurance.
❑ Creates more awareness of correct body positioning.
❑ Strengthens your torso and prepares you for the standing ballet and balance exercises.

Reverse Tabletop

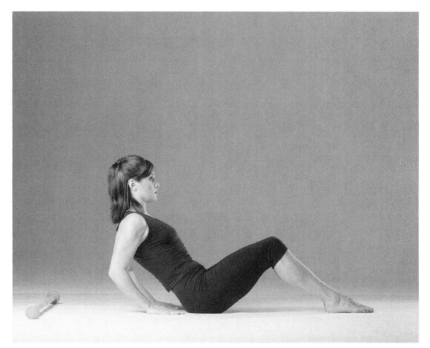

1. Roll onto your bottom. Bend your knees and place the soles of your feet on the floor in parallel. Press your palms into the floor and turn your fingers to face front. Lift your chest. Scoop your abdominals first, then bend your elbows. Firmly press your palms and knuckles into the floor.

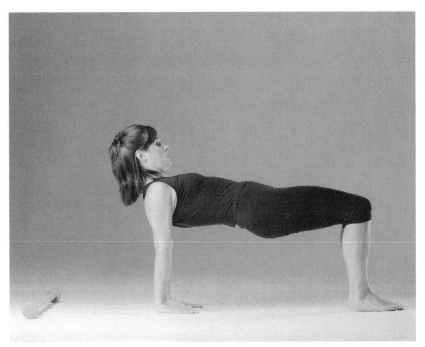

2. Lift your hips and chest up to the ceiling. Keep the knees over your ankles. Look beyond your knees. Hold this position for 15 seconds.

3. Bend your elbows and lower your bottom to come down.

4. Repeat this three times or continue with the next exercise 2 times.

Reverse Plank

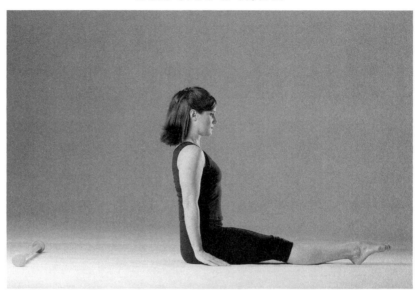

1. Roll onto your bottom. Extend your legs, and pull your inner thighs and feet together tightly. Press your palms into the floor, and turn your fingers to face front. Lift your chest.

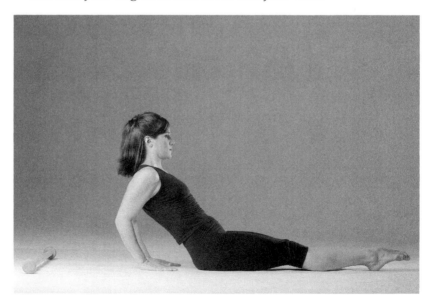

2. Scoop your abdominals first, then bend your elbows. Firmly press your palms and knuckles into the floor. Stretch and point your toes toward the floor.

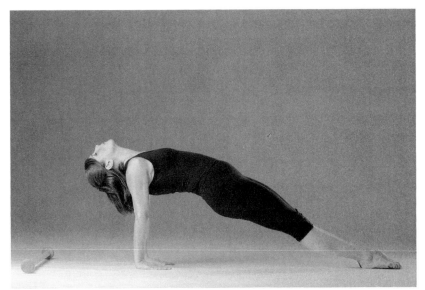

3. Lift your hips and chest up to the ceiling. Point your toes to touch the floor. Keep your inner thighs and buttock muscles engaged. Carefully stretch your neck back with your chin up. Hold this position for 15 seconds.

4. Lower your seat to come down.

5. Sit up tall with your legs fully extended and palms touching the floor.

HELPFUL REMINDERS:

- Keeping your inner thighs together and placing your feet in a parallel position will help you feel balanced and strong as you lift up.
- Take tension out of your wrists by planting your hands into the floor and using the strength of your arms and core muscles.
- Aim your heart and hips up, and reach your legs and head away from your center.

FLOOR BALLET VARIATION: *Point-and-Flex*—

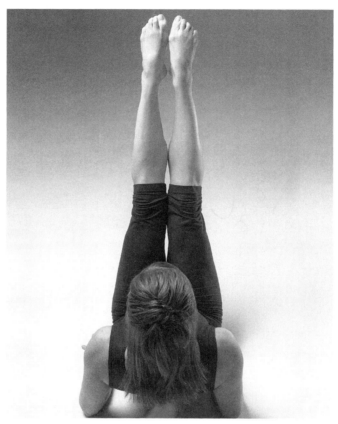

1. Roll onto your forearms, support your upper back, and bring your legs up to a 60-degree angle. In parallel, point your toes.

Parallel

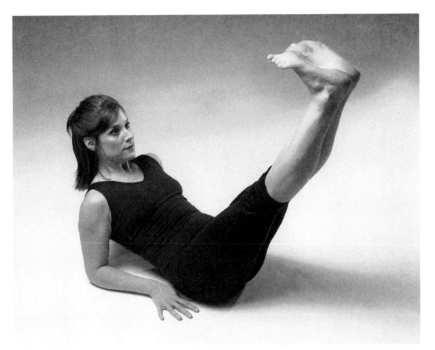

2. Flex your feet, pushing through your heels.

REPEAT 8 TIMES

FLOOR BALLET VARIATION: *Point-and-Flex—*

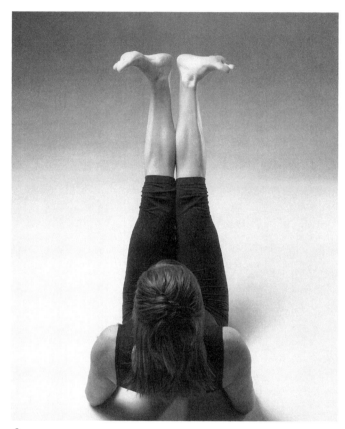

1. Flex your feet and squeeze your inner thighs and buttock muscles. Fan your toes out to your turn-out position. This is first position in ballet.

HELPFUL REMINDER:

- To turn out correctly, the rotation happens from your hip joint rather than your knees or ankles. Do not force your rotation.

First Position

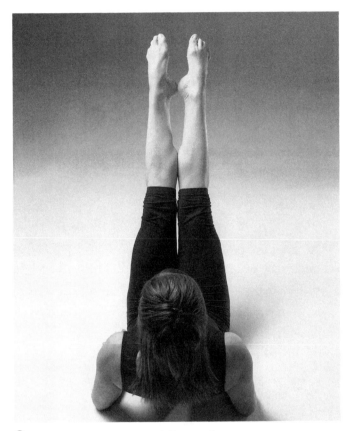

2. Continue to point and flex in first position 8 times.

FLOOR BALLET VARIATION: *Bow-and-Arrow*

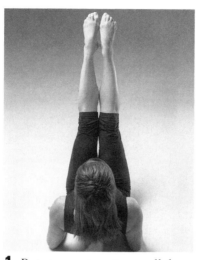

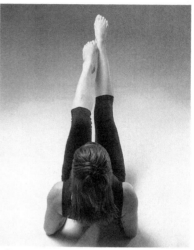

HELPFUL REMINDERS:

- Fully extending your legs and feet will increase the stretch and circulation within your muscles and joints.

- Use the strength of your forearms and correct shoulder placement to avoid collapsing in your chest or shoulder girdle.

1. Point your toes in parallel position. Keeping your right leg stretched and long, engage your abdominals and inner thighs.

2. Draw your left foot to the inside of your right ankle, or to coupé position.

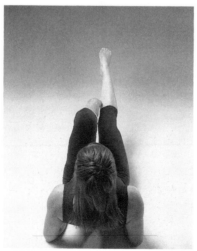

3. Keeping your knee toward your chest, continue to slide your foot up the inside of your right leg, or to passé position. Simultaneously, extend your right leg down toward the floor so your legs split.

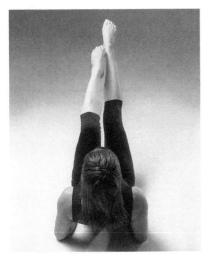

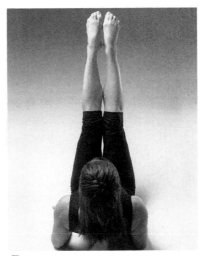

REPEAT 6 TIMES

4. Slide your foot back down the inside of your calf through the coupé position.

5. Stretch the leg to meet your right leg.

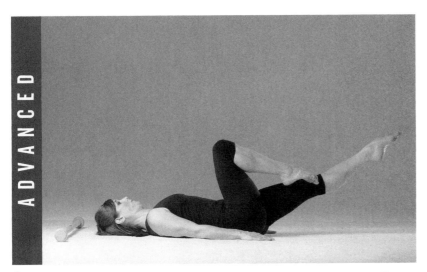

ADVANCED

1. Rather than propping up on your forearms, keep your back flat against the floor while keeping your neck long. While performing these exercises, your back should not arch. Your neck and upper back should also remain firm against the floor.

FLOOR BALLET VARIATION: *Parallel Pliés*

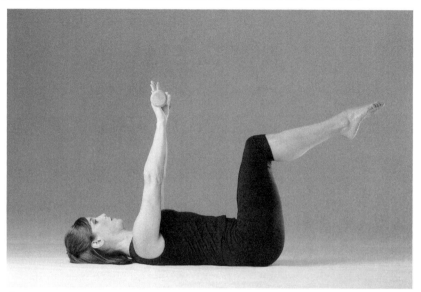

1. Inhale, and lift your feet off the floor, bringing your feet in line with your knees. Your knees should be directly over your hips. Your barre is over your chest.

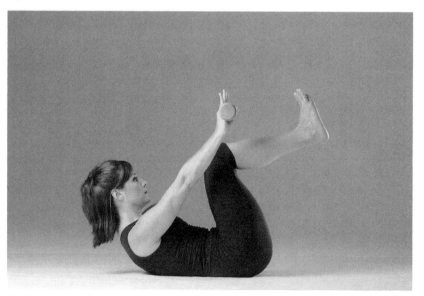

2. Exhale, and lift your head off the floor into your Core Curl-Up position. Flex your feet.

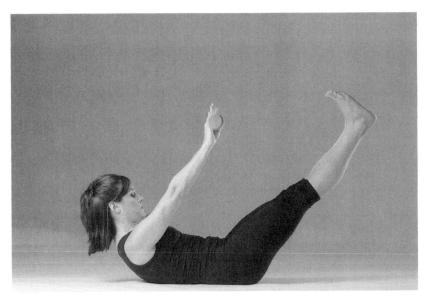

3. On your next exhalation, push your feet away until your legs are
straightened and lengthened.

4. Inhale, and bring the knees back in. Exhale and repeat the pliés
6 times.

FLOOR BALLET VARIATION: *Turned-Out*

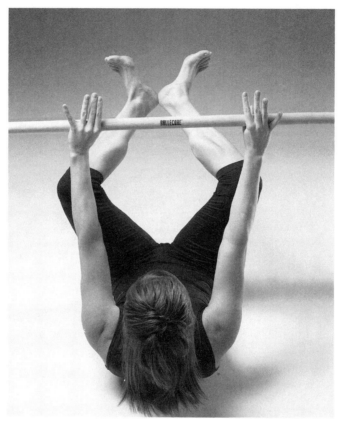

1. Turn your feet out, keeping your heels together and inner thighs rotated. Inhale, and bend your knees, creating a diamond shape between your legs.

HELPFUL REMINDERS:

- In parallel, your knees and inner thighs must stay tightly together as you move in and out.
- As your knees come in, feel your abdominal muscles shrinking smaller into your lower back and waist.
- As your legs extend away from your body, reach out of your hips, creating beautiful extension.
- Lower your head if tension arises within your neck and shoulder area, or place your hands behind your head to support the neck.

(First Position) Pliés

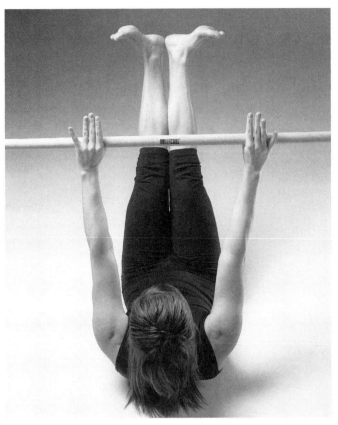

2. Exhale, and send your legs away, pushing directly through your heels.

3. Repeat these pliés 6 times.

4. Bring your knees in slowly, and lower your head and feet to the floor.

FLOOR BALLET VARIATION: *Floor Développés*

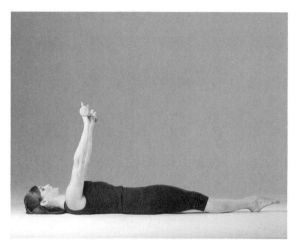

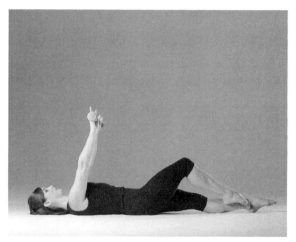

1. Inhale and stretch your body long against the floor. Exhale, bring the barre over your chest, and point your toes.

2. Inhale, in your parallel position, and draw your right foot to the inside of your left ankle, or to coupé.

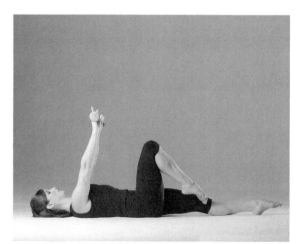

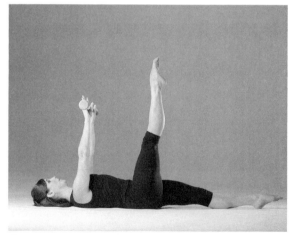

3. Keeping your knee facing directly up to the ceiling, continue to slide your foot up the inside of your left leg, or to passé.

4. Release your foot and extend your leg up to the ceiling, or to développé.

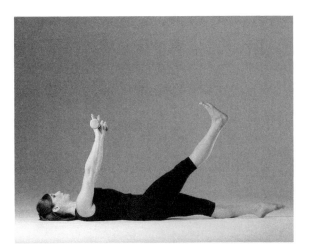

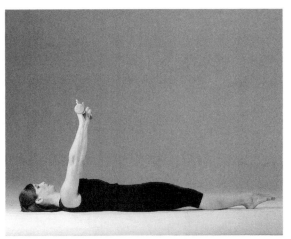

5. Exhale, flex your foot and reach through your heel toward the floor.

6. Stretch your feet and bring your legs together.

REPEAT 3 TIMES

Head Lifted

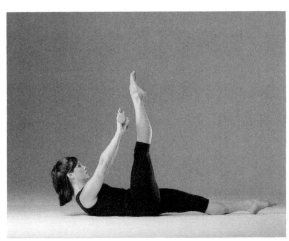

1. Exhale, and lift your head, neck and upper shoulders off the floor to your Core Curl-Up position.

2. Follow steps 2 through 6 above.

3. Repeat 3 times and switch legs.

FLOOR BALLET VARIATION: *Battements*

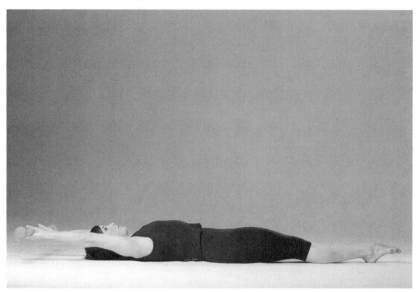

1. Breathe in and out, and stretch your body long against the floor. The barre is overhead, and your toes are pointed.

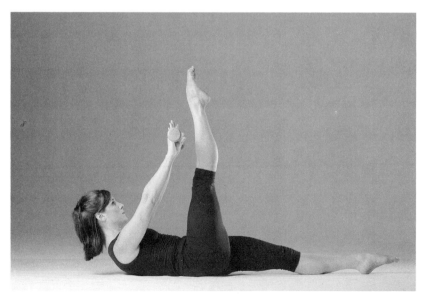

2. Exhale, toss your right leg, or battement, and round your upper back. Your upper body and leg meet directly up toward the ceiling.

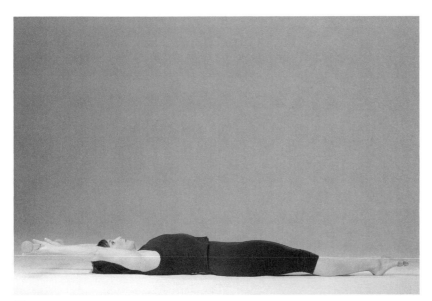

3. Inhale, and your upper back and leg reach down toward the floor simultaneously.

4. Stretch your body long.

5. Exhale and repeat steps 2 through 4 six times.

HELPFUL REMINDERS:

- Your supporting leg (the leg that is not moving) should stay firm against the floor during développés and battements.
- If you find that your leg is coming off the floor, modify by bending this leg and placing the sole of your foot on the floor for additional support.
- Exhale as your leg reaches away from your body.
- Contracting your deep abdominal muscles will protect your back as you lift and lower your working leg.
- Your tailbone never leaves the floor.
- When your head is up, protect your neck by ensuring that you're in the correct Core Curl-Up position.
- Perform the battements slowly; more body control is needed as your limbs meet toward the ceiling.

Roll-Up (Transitional Move)

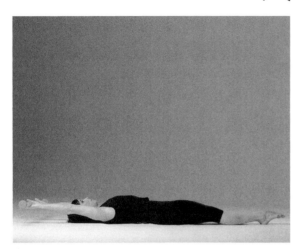

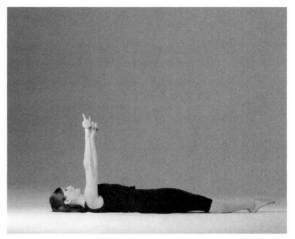

1. Inhale and stretch your arms overhead. Reach for the BalleCore Barre or Band.

2. Exhale and bring the barre up to the ceiling as you engage your ribs and abdominals. Slide your shoulders down.

HELPFUL REMINDERS:

- Keep your breathing fluid and connected to your movements.
- Your rib cage must be closed and your belly must be pulled into the floor to initiate the roll-up.
- Focus on symmetry in your body. Keep your shoulders square, hips in line, and inner thighs activated.
- Use your BalleCore Barre or Band as a resistance tool and guide for your body alignment.

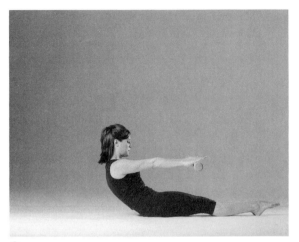

3. Peel off the mat one vertebra at a time, with your arms at chest level.

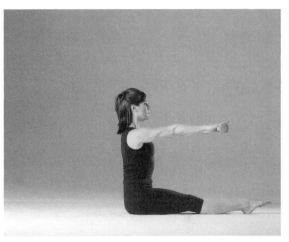

4. Continue to roll up until you are sitting up tall.

Half Roll-up

If you are having difficulty rolling off the mat, try bending your knees and follow steps 1 through 4.

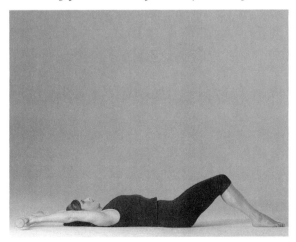

Teaser Variation

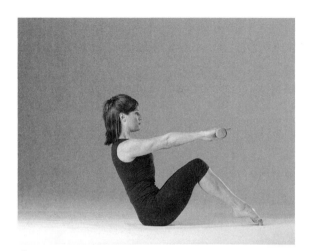

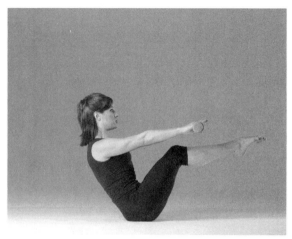

1. Sitting up tall, pull your legs together and point your toes. Lift off your seat by engaging your buttock muscles. Slide your knees in toward your chest while keeping your toes pointed. Scoop out your abdominal muscles and tilt back between your sitting bones and tailbone.

2. Test your balance by slowly lifting your toes off the floor. Continue to balance and raise your feet so your ankles are in line with your knees.

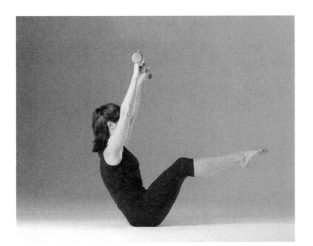

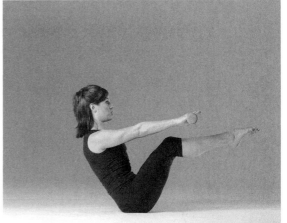

3. Inhale and slowly lift your arms up.

4. Exhale and lower your arms back to chest level.

5. Repeat raising the barre (steps 3 and 4) 4 times.

(continued on next page)

Teaser Variation (continued)

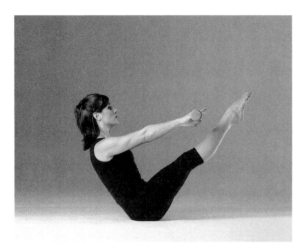

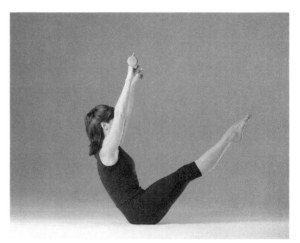

6. Extend both legs, keeping your inner thighs and knees connected.

7. Inhale and raise the barre overhead. Exhale and lower your barre back to chest level.

HELPFUL REMINDERS:

- Although the Teaser requires strong core muscles, these steps guide you from easy to more challenging positions to help you build strength and endurance.

- Steps 6 and 7 are more advanced positions with straight legs. You can go directly from step 4 to step 8 to the finish.

- The inner thighs and knees must always be seamed together in order to work the body in symmetry.

- Take weight out of your lower back by gently squeezing your buttock muscles and pulling your abdominal muscles inward and up.

- As you lift the BalleCore Barre overhead, bring it up slowly. The barre never goes behind your ears.

- Breathe in and out steadily and fluidly.

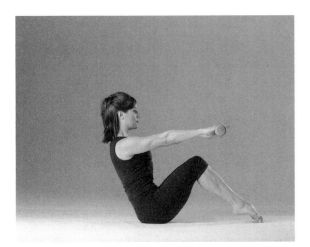

8. Lower both feet to the floor, keeping your toes pointed with your heels lifted off the floor.

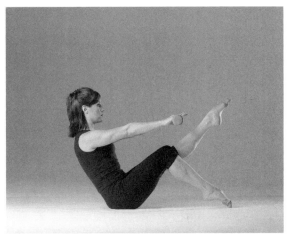

9. Extend your left leg and lower. Your knees are touching.

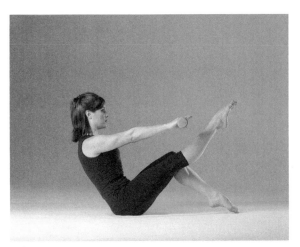

10. Extend your right leg and lower. Your knees are touching.

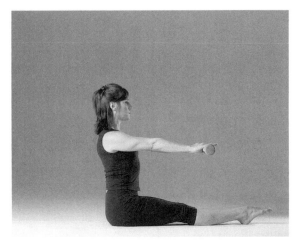

11. Sit up tall, reaching your legs out.

12. Repeat 2 times, breathing mindfully throughout the steps.

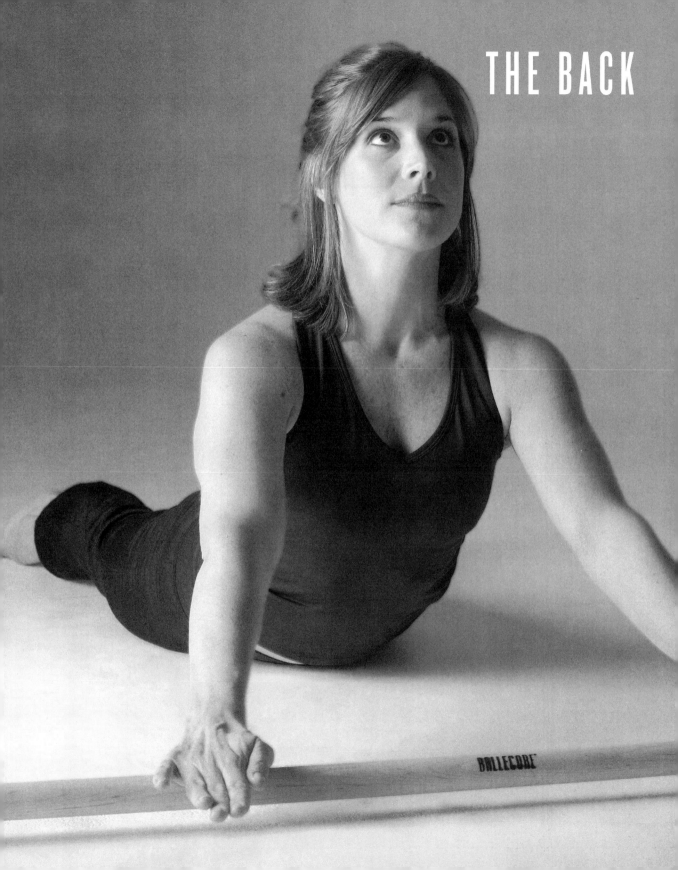

THE BACK

The Back

Keeping the spine supple and strong is the key to youthfulness. It will also make your daily activities feel much easier and more stress-free. I will take you through some gentle back-strengthening exercises and some that will require more muscular strength. Opening up areas in the back, releasing unwanted tension in the neck and shoulders, promotes better posture and allows more freedom for your body to move with grace and ease.

Benefits:

❑ Creates a more flexible spine.

❑ Strengthens the back and improves posture.

❑ Restores balance in the musculature.

❑ Frees restricted breathing and increases circulation.

COBRA VARIATION: *Cobra with Pulses*

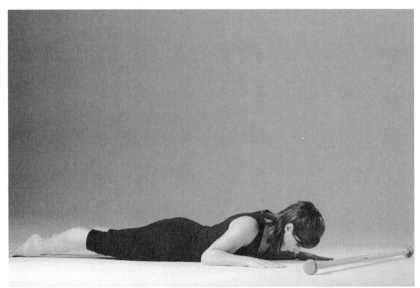

1. Lie facedown with your hips and pelvis supported by pulling your abdominal muscles up into your back. Place your hands and palms down at your sides. Spread your fingers by the sides of your shoulders. Stretch your legs long with the tops of the thighs parallel to the floor.

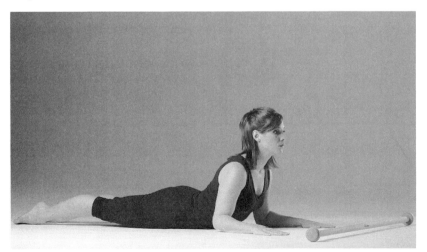

2. Inhale, and firmly press your palms and forearms into the floor as you lift your chest up and roll your shoulders back. Tighten your buttock muscles keeping the tops of your feet on the floor.

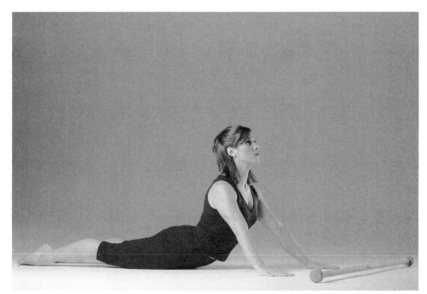

3. Continue lifting your chest and trunk until your arms are straightened. Keep your neck long. Hold this position for a few seconds.

4. Repeat the action of pumping your arms up and halfway down 4 times. Breathe naturally.

5. Exhale and lower your trunk, slowly. Keep your elbows close to your sides.

COBRA VARIATION: *Cobra Roll*

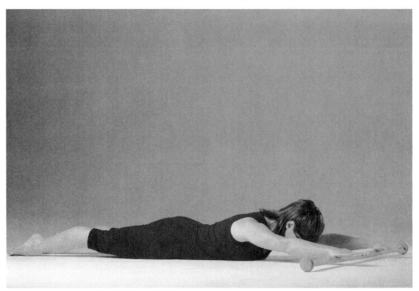

1. Lie facedown with your hips and pelvis supported by pulling your abdominal muscles up into your back. Stretch your arms out and place your hands and palms firmly on the BalleCore Barre. Stretch your legs long, with the tops of your thighs parallel to the floor.

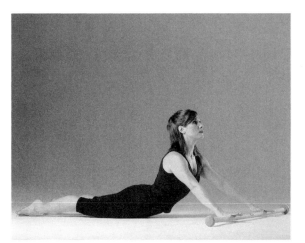 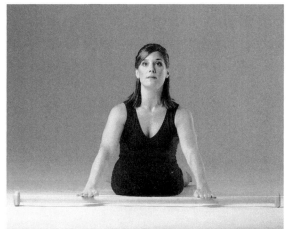

2. Inhale, tighten your buttock muscles, and lift your chest as you roll the barre toward your body. Keep the thighs and tops of your feet firmly against the floor. Hold the position for a few seconds.

3. Exhale, and with control roll the barre away from your body. Stretch your body long.

REPEAT 4 TIMES

COBRA VARIATION: *Cobra Rocking*

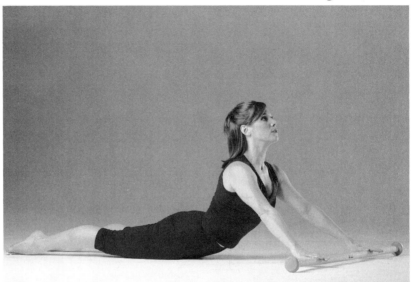

1. Inhale, and lift your chest as you roll the barre toward your body. Keep your thighs, your buttocks, and the tops of your feet firmly against the floor. Hold your position for two seconds.

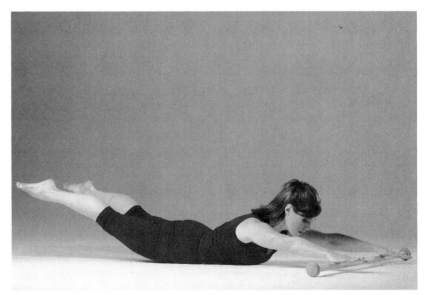

2. Exhale, press your hands into the barre, and rock forward. Lift your legs off the floor.

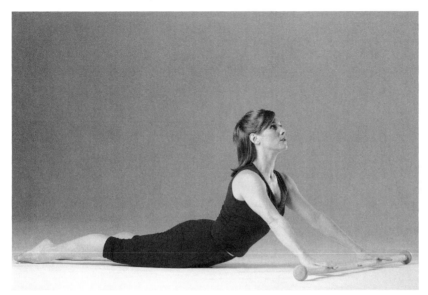

3. Inhale, roll the barre toward you, and lift your chest up.

4. Rock back and forth 4 times.

5. Exhale, and roll back down slowly.

6. Stretch your body long.

HELPFUL REMINDERS:

- The Cobra Rolls and Rocking can be added to the Pulses as your back becomes stronger and more flexible.

- Keep the tops of your feet and thighs firmly against the floor throughout, to avoid overusing your buttock muscles and straining your lower back.

- Press against the floor to increase the intensity of the stretch in your upper back.

- As you raise your chest, feel your sternum lifting up while your shoulders roll back.

- Keep your neck in line with your spine as you lift.

Star Fish

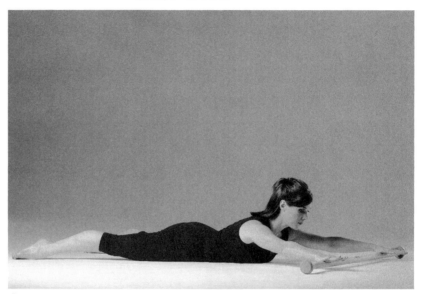

1. Lying facedown, extend your arms and legs into a small V position 3 to 4 inches outside your shoulders and hips. Place your hands and palms firmly on the BalleCore Barre or floor. Support your hips and pelvis by pulling your abdominal muscles up into your back. Stretch your legs long, with the tops of your thighs slightly turned out on the floor; inhale.

2. Exhale, and lift your right leg and left arm. Hold the position for a few seconds.

HELPFUL REMINDERS:

- Your legs and arms should be about 3 or 4 inches outside the shoulder girdle and hip socket to work specific muscles in the back and buttocks.

- Activate your abdominal muscles and rib cage while your hips stay against the floor. This allows your limbs to move freely.

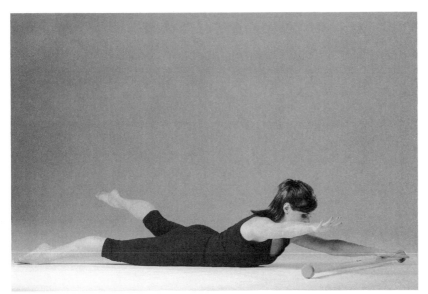

3. Inhale, and alternate lifting your left leg and right arm. Hold the position for a few seconds.

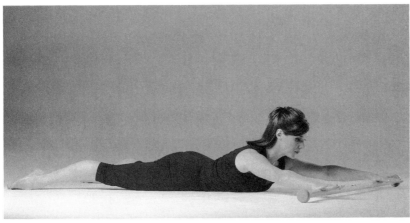

4. Repeat this action, moving your opposite legs and arms quicker for 6 repetitions. Breathe in and out. Lower your legs and stretch your arms long.

PRONE BALLET VARIATION:

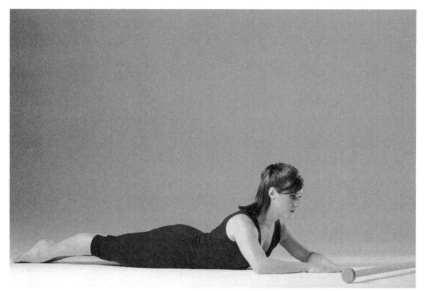

1. On your stomach, bring your arms to a triangle position in front of your upper body. Your chest and upper back are lifted and stabilized. Your fingertips are together, and your elbows are wide. Your hips and pelvis are supported as you pull your abdominal muscles up into your back. Stretch your legs and feet long, with the tops of the thighs parallel to the floor.

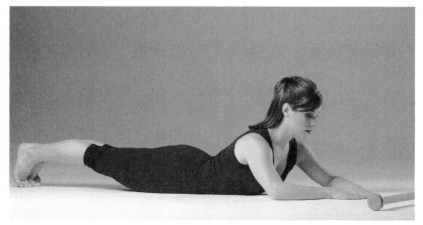

2. Curl your toes under, or to demi-pointe position. Now flex your feet, firmly push through your heels, and straighten your legs.

Flex—Point—Leg Extension

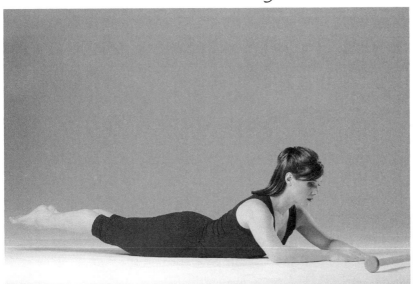

3. Point your toes, stretch your legs, and lift your knees off
the floor.

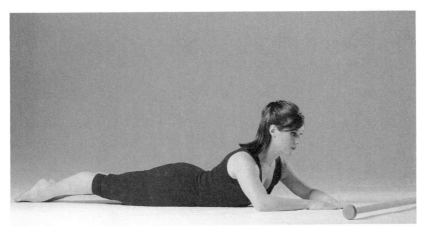

4. Slowly lower your legs.

REPEAT 4 TIMES

PRONE BALLET VARIATION: *Floor Dancer's Pose*

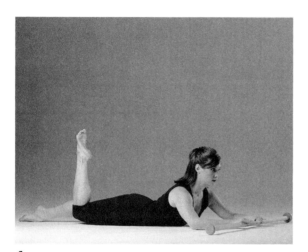

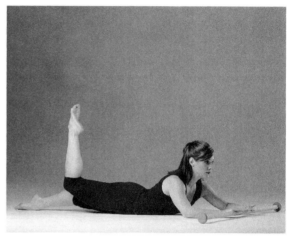

1. On your stomach, bring your arms to a triangle position in front of your upper body. Your chest and upper back are lifted. Your fingertips are together, and your elbows are wide. Protect your lower back by pulling your abdominal muscles up into your back. Stretch your legs and feet long, with the tops of your thighs parallel to the floor. Bend your right knee as you firmly press your thighs into the floor.

2. Lift your knee off the floor, keeping your hip on the floor and your leg at a right angle. Your knee is still in line with your hip bone.

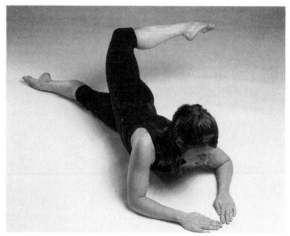

3. Lift your right hip and thigh off the floor. Aim your toes toward the left side. Reach and touch the floor with your foot on your left side, keeping your leg bent (to attitude position) and your thigh lengthened.

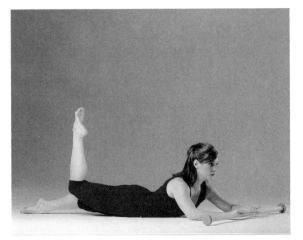 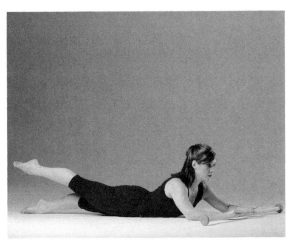

4. Bring your thigh back so your hip touches the floor. Stretch your leg out.

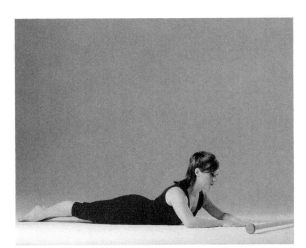

HELPFUL REMINDERS:

- Use the strength of your forearms and shoulders to help brace your upper back.

- Keep your legs, buttocks, and abdominal muscles engaged as you lift over to stretch and lengthen the lumbar spine.

- The front of your thigh should be long as you cross it over.

5. Lower your foot.

6. Repeat 3 times and switch to the other leg.

Diagonal Reaches

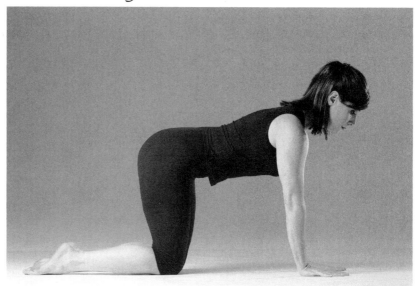

- To take pressure out of your knees and wrists, your trunk muscles must be engaged.

- As you move your limbs horizontal, then back to your vertical position, keep your hips down.

- Practice lifting and lowering your limbs up and down before stretching them to the side. Coordination and balance are tested here.

1. Kneel with your hands on the floor directly under your shoulders and your knees underneath your hip bones. Keep your neck long and stomach and ribs pulled in.

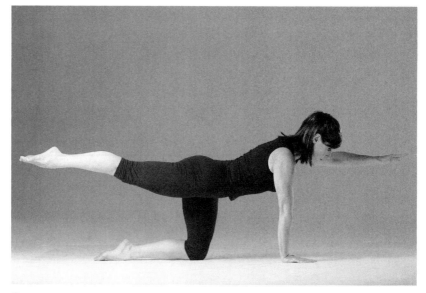

2. Inhale, and lift your right leg and left arm off the floor so that your body is in a straight line from your toes to your fingertips.

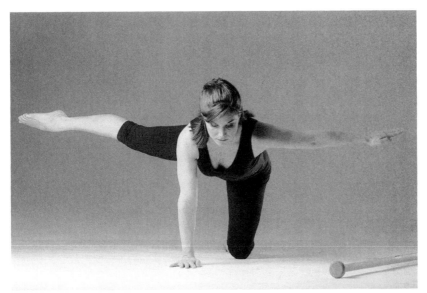

3. Exhale, and reach your leg and arm simultaneously out to the side.

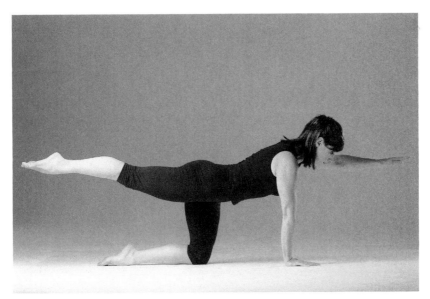

4. Inhale, then bring your leg and arm back in line so that your body is in a straight line.

5. Repeat 4 times on each side.

Plank Position Combination

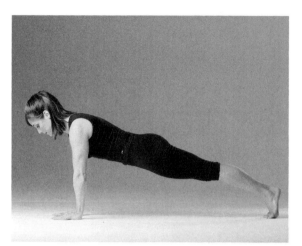

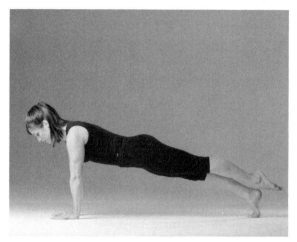

1. Kneel with your hands on the floor directly under your shoulders. Place your knees underneath your hip bones. Keep your neck long and your stomach and ribs pulled in. Extend both legs and pull your inner thighs together tightly. Push through both heels.

2. Take your left foot off the floor and point your toes.

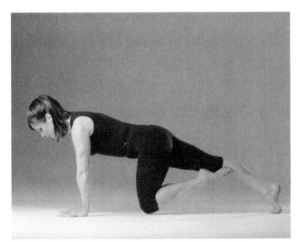

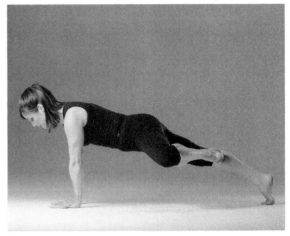

3. Starting at the ankle, slide your left foot up the inside of your right leg, or to coupé. Continue sliding your foot up your inner thigh to the knee, or to passé.

4. Rotate your knee to turn out.

5. Turn your left knee back to parallel, in passé.

(continued on next page)

Plank Position Combination (continued)

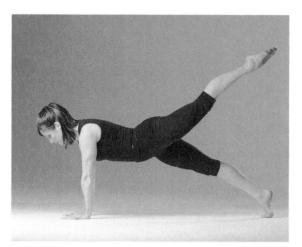

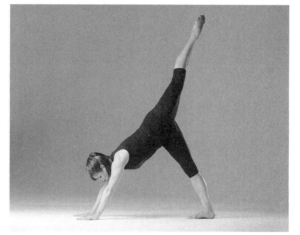

6. Slide your left leg down the inside of your right leg, to meet your right leg with your foot pointed. Lift your left leg up, as high as possible, while staying in your Plank Position.

7. In Plank, shift your sitting bones and buttocks up to the ceiling and press your hands firmly into the floor. Allow your leg to float up high (or to penché), creating a long diagonal line from your hands to your toes. Expand your torso and allow your neck to relax. Keep your right foot flat on the floor.

8. Engaging your center, shift your left leg back to Plank Position, placing your hands under your shoulder and heels, reaching away. Bend your knees, then shift your seat back over the soles of your feet. Stretch your arms in front of your body.

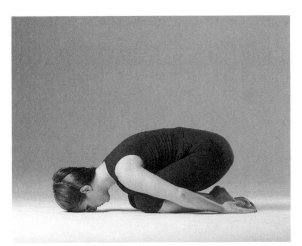

9. Slowly bring your arms around to your heels, and slow down your breathing. Relax in Child's Pose.

10. Repeat this combination 2 times on each leg.

HELPFUL REMINDERS:

- Engage your abdominal muscles by drawing them up toward your spine.

- Feel the front of your body pulling up into your back.

- Distribute your weight evenly between your hands and fingers. This will take unnecessary pressure out of your wrists, and send energy and power up your arms and shoulders.

- Do not arch your back or tuck your chin under.

- In your resting position, allow your physical body to relax. Focus inward and breathe normally.

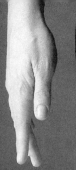

STANDING BALLET

Standing Ballet

You don't need to be a prima ballerina to enjoy the results of what basic ballet can do for the body and soul. This series of exercises and positions is a friendly introduction to the beginner who has never learned the basics in a traditional ballet class. I have chosen just a few to share with you because of their universal physical benefits.

In this section, I will also ask you to test your balance by lifting your heels. This is an easy way to gauge your sense of control.

The second important aspect of this section is the use of arms. We continuously want to challenge our bodies as we strive to improve our appearance. Therefore, I have introduced specific arm movements that coordinate with what you're doing with the lower half of your body. These arm movements are called port de bras, which translates from the French as "carriage of the arms." Port de bras helps you strengthen your upper back and torso. Working your arms through port de bras while also exercising the legs create a more challenging exercise experience. Incorporating port de bras throughout the workout is a unique way to increase range of motion in tight shoulders, enhance the shape of the shoulders and arms, and improve coordination. You will begin to feel just how natural new movements become, as if you're an experienced dancer. Coordination and mental focus are required as you work the arms and legs in these different positions. With practice, you will learn to perform these exercises like a dancer, with elegance and grace, by emphasizing gorgeous lines.

Benefits:

- ❑ Challenges and improves balance as you move in space.
- ❑ Sculpts the quadriceps and calves, and strengthens the ankles.
- ❑ Emphasizes core stabilization and posture.

PROPER PARALLEL STANCE

1. Stand with your feet together and in parallel.

2. Distribute your weight evenly among the heels, arches, and balls of your feet.

3. Engage your inner thighs and groin. Draw your thigh muscles upward, taking pressure off your kneecaps.

4. Lift your abdominal muscles up toward your back to support your frame.

5. Relax your tailbone so it is parallel to the floor.

6. Reach your arms down toward the floor.

7. Extend your spine up and open your chest.

8. Drop your shoulders and lengthen your neck, feeling a lift through the crown of your head.

Positions of the BalleCore Barre

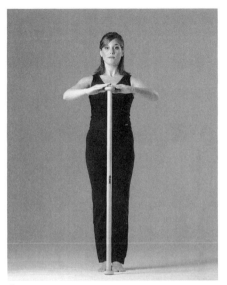

1. Place the barre on the floor, directly in front of the center of your body. Your arms are slightly curved.

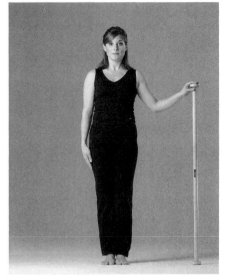

2. Place the barre at your side, slightly in front of your shoulder.

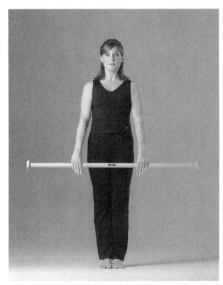

3. Place the barre in both hands directly in front of your thighs.

(continued on next page)

Positions of the BalleCore Barre (continued)

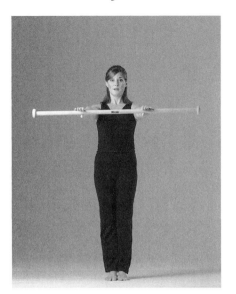 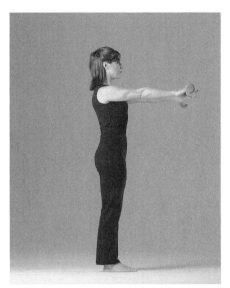

4. Place the barre horizontally in front of your chest.

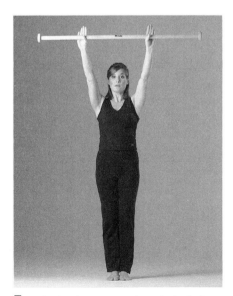

5. Lift the barre overhead slightly in front of your shoulders.

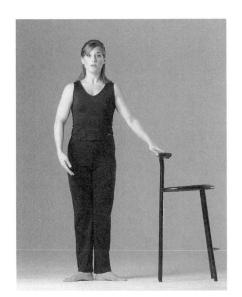 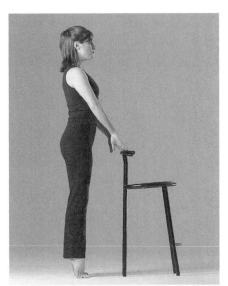

6. If you are using a chair, step approximately 6 inches away from it and rest your fingers on the chair for balance.

Pilates V Position Balance

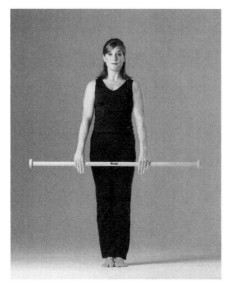 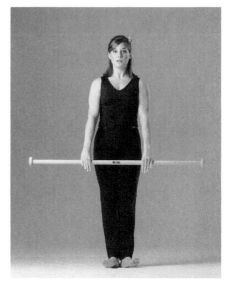

1. Stand tall in your parallel position with the barre at your hips.

2. Rotate your legs and feet into a small V position. Tighten your inner thighs.

HELPFUL REMINDERS:

- As you relevé, continue to pull up and lengthen the front of your body to engage your inner abdominal muscles. Narrow the pelvis.

- If your heels come apart, your V is too wide.

- As you carry the barre up and down, move it slowly and breathe with fluidity.

- Inner focus is required for balance.

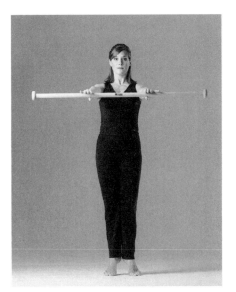 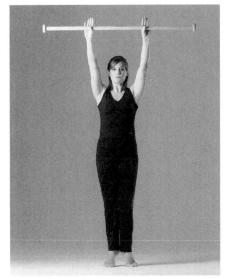

3. Rise up to relevé, keeping your heels together. Lift the barre and hold it at chest level.

4. Inhale, and raise the barre overhead, while at the same time drawing your shoulder blades down.

5. Exhale, lower the barre to chest level, and hold.

6. Continue lowering the barre down to your hips, and lower your heels. Repeat steps 3–6 four times.

PARALLEL VARIATION: *Relevés*

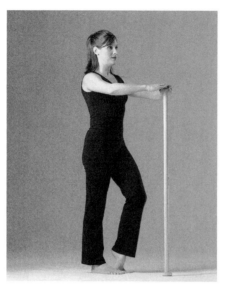

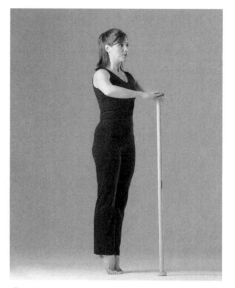

1. Lift your left heel up as you place weight on the ball of your foot.

2. Rise up and lift both heels and arches off the floor, pressing your inner thighs together, to relevé.

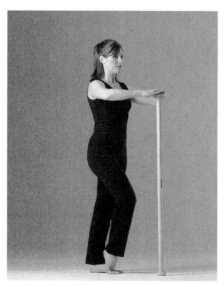

3. Switch, lowering your left heel and lifting your right heel.

4. Lift up and lower to relevé 8 times. Both heels lift off the floor, pressing your inner thighs together.

and Pliés

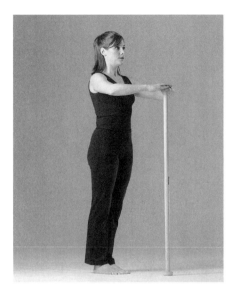

5. Straighten both legs.

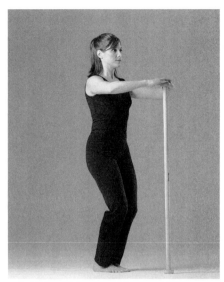

6. Bend your knees, or demi-plié.

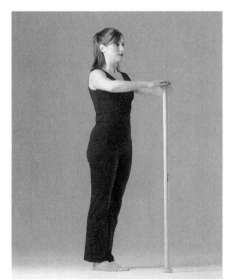

7. Straighten both legs.

8. Plié and straighten 8 times. Keep feet flat on the floor, pressing your inner thighs together.

HELPFUL REMINDERS:

- Keep your body weight centered as you transfer from foot to foot.
- As your heels lift, your weight is on the base of your big and second toes and on the balls of your feet.
- The spine is lengthened, keeping the front of your body long.
- While standing, activate your thigh muscles and pelvic floor muscles by pulling the upper thigh, inner thigh, and buttock muscles together.

TURN-OUT (FIRST POSITION) VARIATION: *Relevés*

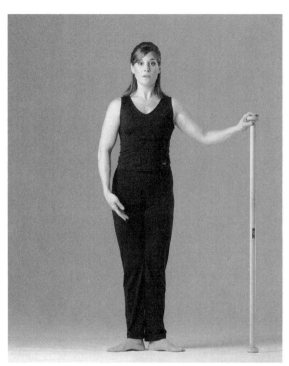 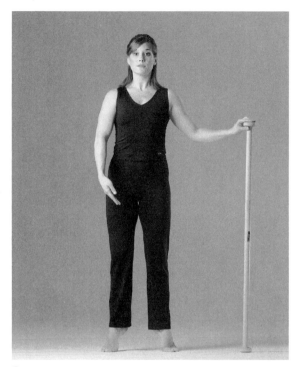

1. Standing in your parallel position, rotate your legs and knees and fan your toes outward, within the hips. This is first position in ballet.

2. Lift your heels and arches, or relevé, as you push into the balls of your feet.

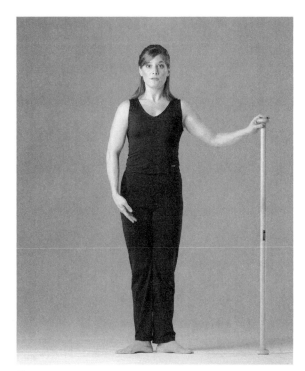

3. Slowly lower your heels, keeping your inner thighs engaged and chest lifted.

4. Return to your turn-out position and repeat 8 times.

TURN-OUT (FIRST POSITION) VARIATION:

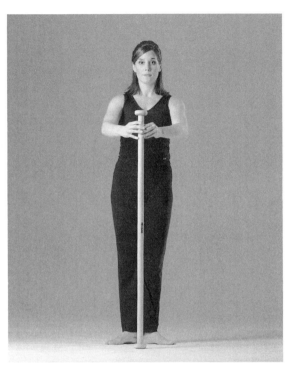

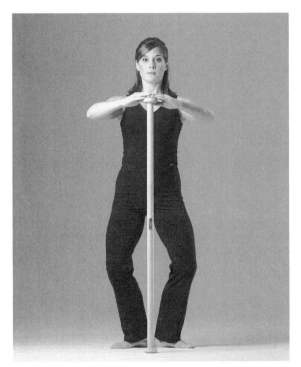

1. Place your barre so it is in front of your body, long.

2. Bend the knees, or demi-plié, keeping your heels down and knees over the toes.

Plié—Relevé—Balance

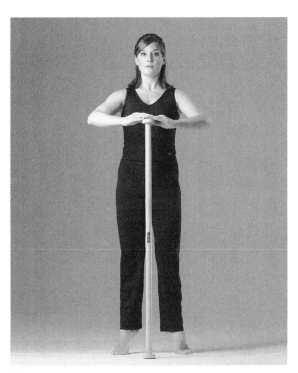

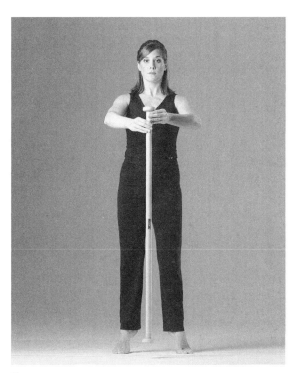

3. Push off the floor, and straighten your legs and lift your heels to relevé.

4. Lower your heels and bend your knees to demi-plié.

5. Push off the floor, and straighten your legs and lift your heels to relevé. Repeat plié-relevé six times.

6. Lift your heels to relevé, and, with mental focus, lift your barre off the floor two inches. Test your balance for several seconds.

TURN-OUT (FIRST POSITION) VARIATION:

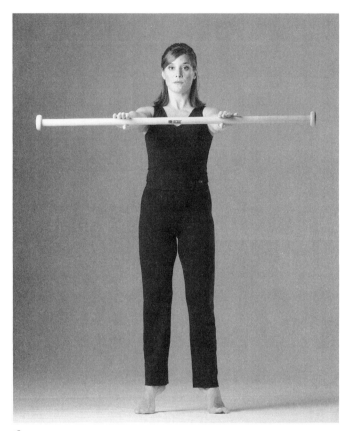

1. Hold the barre directly in front of your chest with your arms and fingers stretched long. Hold this position 10–30 seconds.

Balance Test with the BalleCore Barre Horizontal

HELPFUL REMINDERS:

- To find your natural turn-out position, engage your inner thigh and buttock muscles and rotate your toes outward, so that your knees are directly over your toes. This action begins at your hip socket.

- Always lift the weight of your body off the legs with pliés. Relax your knee joints.

- Pull in your abdominal muscles and keep your lower spine lengthened so that you are not tucking or arching.

- Resist the floor as you lower your heels with ease.

Tendu to the Side

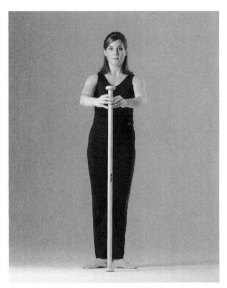 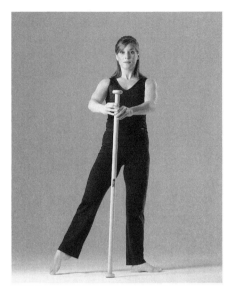

1. Stand tall in your turn-out position, or first position.

2. Shift your weight slightly to your left foot as your right heel reaches to the side. Fully point your toes and lift your arch.

HELPFUL REMINDERS:

- Feel the stretch down your leg, starting with your thighs, down to your ankles, and out through the toes.
- Practice your balance as you shift your weight from side to side. Keep your center strong and engaged.
- Always begin stretching by leading with your heel, and then fully extend your foot.
- As you tendu to the side, keep your leg slightly in front of your hip, keeping your hips square and posture correct.

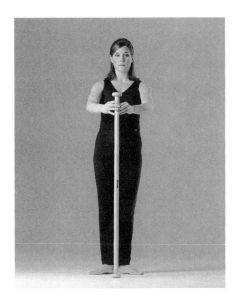

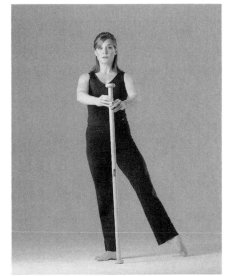

3. Bring the right foot back to the starting position, or first position.

4. Repeat steps 1 through 3 six times.

5. Shift your weight slightly to your right foot as your left heel reaches to the side. Fully point your toes and lift the arch.

6. Repeat on the other side 6 times.

SECOND POSITION VARIATION: *Grand Pliés*

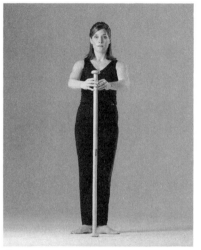 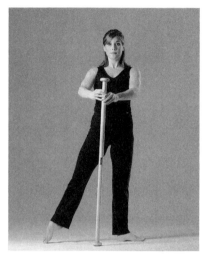

1. In your first position, stretch your right foot to the side to tendu.

HELPFUL REMINDERS:

- Always lift the weight of your body off the legs with pliés. Relax your knee joints.
- Always draw your abdominal muscles up and in, and lengthen the back by drawing your tailbone down and lifting your chest.
- Keep equal weight on both feet, and activate your thighs.
- Pull upward as you bend deeply, taking unnecessary weight off your knees.

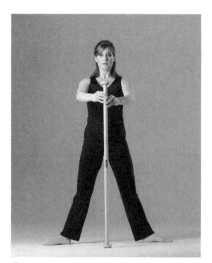 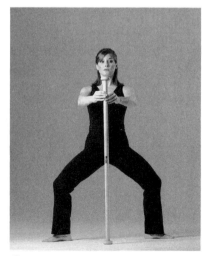

2. Walk your left foot out so your legs are 18 to 24 inches wide. This is second position in ballet.

3. Bend your knees to plié.

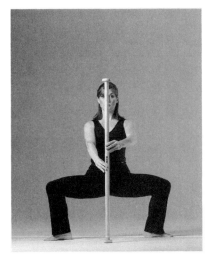

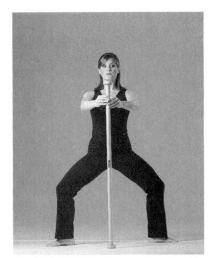

REPEAT 2 TIMES

4. Continue to bend your knees and walk your hands down the BalleCore Barre to deepen your stretch. This is your grand plié.

5. Passing through your plié, straighten your legs.

SECOND POSITION VARIATION: *The Barre Horizontal*

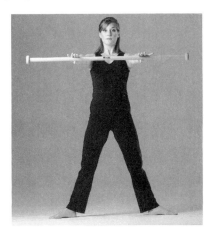

1. Follow the steps above, but place the barre in front of your chest.

SECOND POSITION VARIATION: *Grand Pliés*

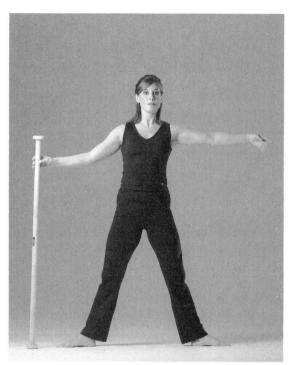

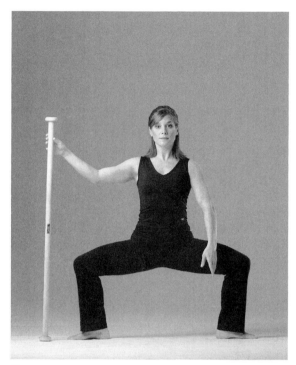

1. Hold your barre or chair to the side in second position, with your legs 18 inches apart. Extend and slightly round your left arm and fingers to the side, just below shoulder level. Your palm faces front, and your wrist and fingers complete the curve of the arm.

2. Plié, and continue to bend your knees deeper into your grand plié. Gracefully lower your left arm down to your hip.

with Port de Bras

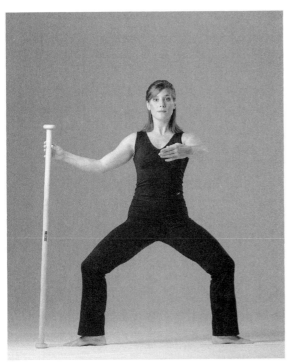

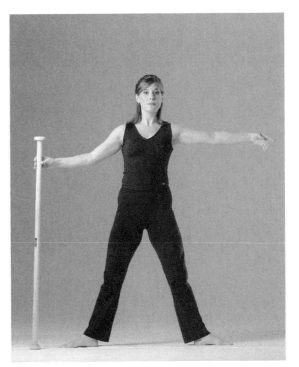

3. Come up slowly to your demi-plié, or small plié, bringing your arm to chest height in front.

4. Straighten your legs and extend your arm back to your side.

5. Repeat 2 times and switch arms.

HELPFUL REMINDERS:

- Press your thighs back as you bend deeply.
- Allow your tailbone to drop as you lift your abdominal muscles.
- Move your arms and legs simultaneously, working on coordination.
- Your arms should be working in a continuous, flowing manner, and should appear relaxed.
- Follow the line of your arm with your fingers flowing in the same direction, creating beautiful lines.
- Keep the integrity of your upper back position as you move your arms through port de bras.
- Port de bras sculpt your arms.

SECOND POSITION VARIATION: *Dégagé—*

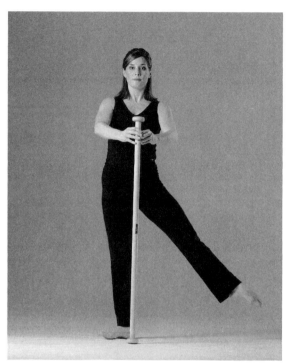

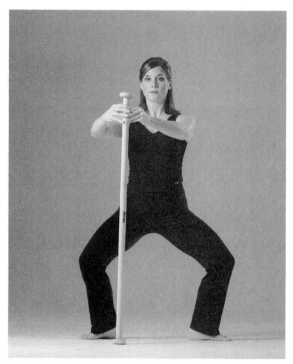

1. In your first position, stretch and brush your left leg outward through your pointe tendu position. Lift your toes from the floor, to dégagé.

2. Firmly lower your left foot and bend your knees wide so your legs are 18 inches apart. This is plié in second position.

Second Position Plié—Balance

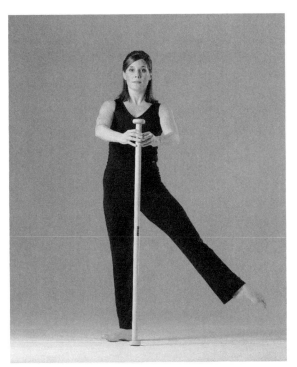

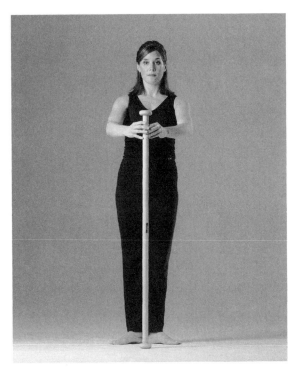

3. Shift your body weight to your right leg as your left leg pushes off the floor back to dégagé. Hold your leg in dégagé for a split second.

4. Repeat steps 2 and 3 six times.

5. Straighten your legs, stretch your left leg, and close to first position.

HELPFUL REMINDERS:

- Dégagés are strong and energetic moves that require the legs and buttocks to be working.
- As you brush your right foot to dégagé, transfer your body weight slightly to the left so you have balance.
- Your inner thighs must be engaged as your leg brushes outward.
- Feel your feet completely stretched in the air and firmly planted into the floor as you plié.
- To make this exercise more advanced, hold the barre in front of your chest horizontally.

SECOND POSITION VARIATION: *Around the World*

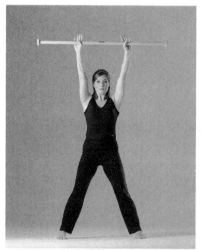

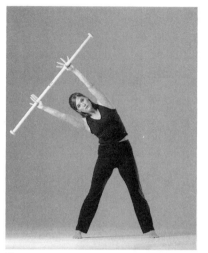

1. In your second position, turn your toes and knees to face front in parallel. Lift your barre or band overhead, keeping your shoulders down.

2. Bend to your right, or cambré to the side, reaching up and then over.

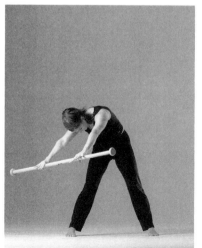

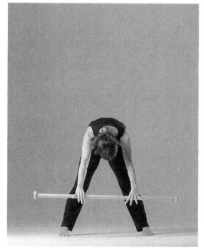

3. Round your trunk forward, allowing your head, neck, and shoulders to stretch. Keep your abdominal muscles engaged.

4. Continue to round over to the center of your body, and cambré forward.

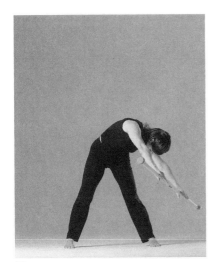

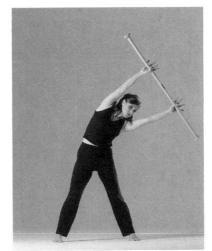

5. Round your trunk over to your left, allowing your head, neck, and shoulders to stretch.

6. Bend to your left, or cambré to the side, reaching up and then over.

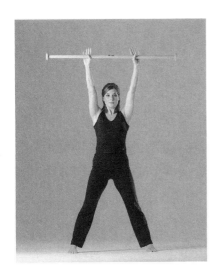

7. Reach up to the ceiling, lengthening your body straight.

8. Repeat all steps 2 times in each direction.

Around the World—with BalleCore Band

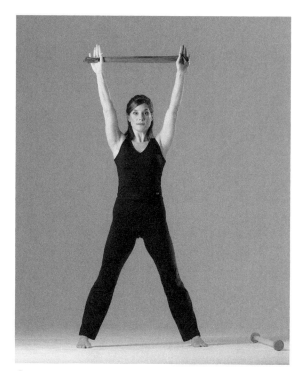 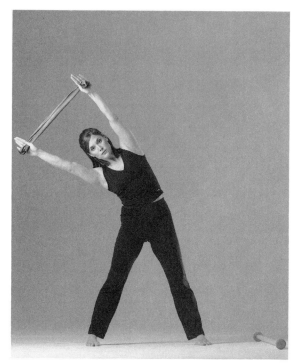

1. Double up your band and hold it so it has resistance, working your arms and shoulders.

HELPFUL REMINDERS:

- Firmly ground your feet into the floor before you begin the exercise.

- Your legs and core muscles must be activated throughout.

- Breathe mindfully as you rotate and circle your torso.

- Hold the barre or band as wide as your shoulders.

- Overbending to the side will make your ribs collapse.

Standing Torso Stretch

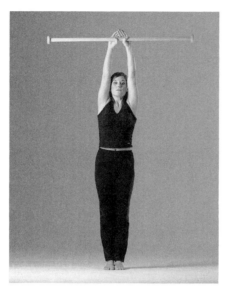 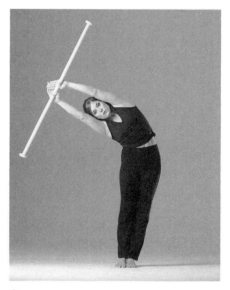

1. Stand in parallel position with your hands close together over the barre. Inhale, and lift the barre overhead, bringing your arms to your ears. Exhale.

2. Inhale, and stretch over to your right, keeping your arms to your ears and your inner thighs connected.

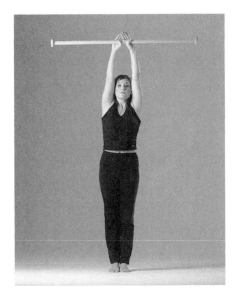

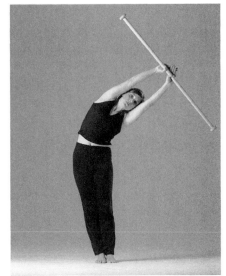

3. Exhale, straighten up, and reach high.

4. Inhale, and stretch over to your left, keeping your arms to your ears and your inner thighs connected.

(continued on next page)

Standing Torso Stretch (continued)

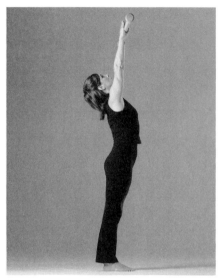

5. Exhale, straighten up, and reach high.

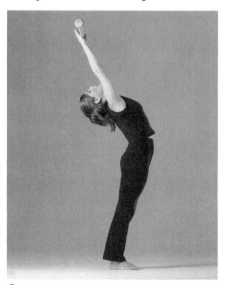

6. Inhale, and continue to reach the barre overhead and allow your chest to open up and bend. Press your hips forward, and tighten your inner thighs.

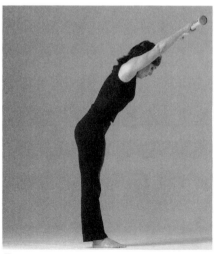

7. Inhale, scoop your abdominals, and stretch forward, bending at your hips.

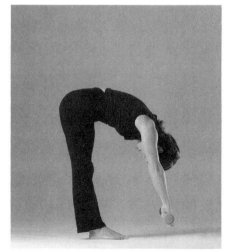

8. Allow your head, shoulders, and entire spine to hang down. Draw the front of your thighs up out of your knees.

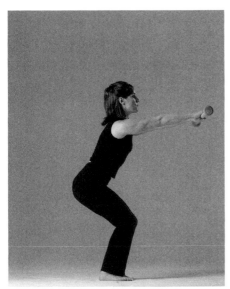

9. Sit back, keeping your knees connected as you bend into Chair Pose. Keep your weight in the balls, arches, and heels of your feet. Lift your chest and lower your tailbone.

10. Straighten your legs to finish.

HELPFUL REMINDERS:

- Inhale deeply as you stretch upward. Exhale deeply as you bend to your sides. Exhale deeply as you stretch forward.

- Keep your legs engaged, and lengthen your spine by drawing your tailbone down.

- Protect your lower back by pulling your abdominals inward and up to bend backward.

- In Chair Pose, drop your buttocks and tailbone. Your arms should be stretched at chest level and parallel to the floor.

REPEAT 2 TIMES

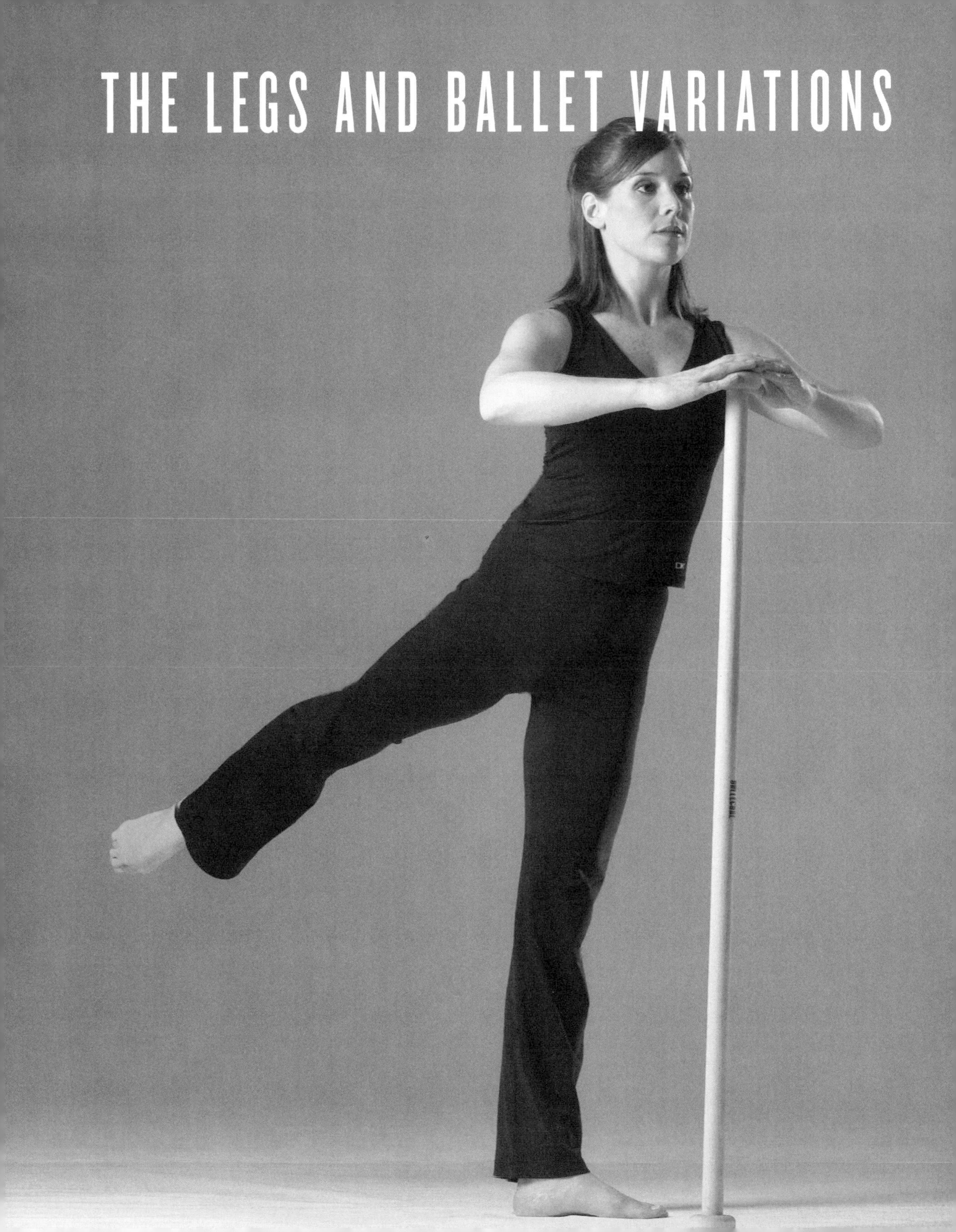

The Legs and Ballet Variations

Building strength and muscle tone in the legs, hips, and gluteals is key to endurance and power in the lower body. Don't worry that you'll develop bulky muscles; the results will be softly sculpted and toned because you are using the weight of your own body rather than traditional heavy weights and machines. Caring for every part of your body and at every level from the inside out will allow your body to explore more complex movements. Let's take the next step, combining longer exercise variations and learning to exercise on one leg.

Benefits:

❑ Builds lower body strength.
❑ Challenges core stability and symmetry in the body.
❑ Tests endurance, concentration, and control.

Rond de Jambe Series

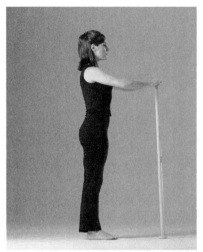

1. Stand in parallel position with your barre in the center of your body.

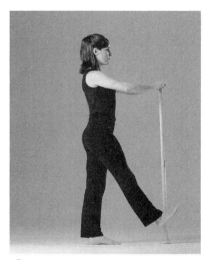

2. Slightly shift your weight to your left foot as you lift your right leg to the front, leading with your heel. Flex your right foot.

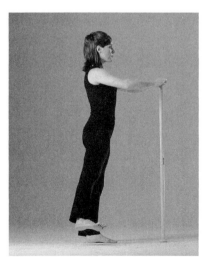

3. Leading with your outer heel, continue to make a circular movement and bring the leg directly to your side.

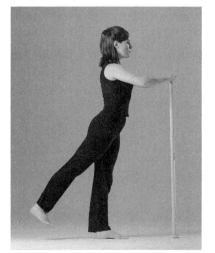

4. Circle the leg to the back, directly behind you, and face your toes front.

5. Slide your foot close in parallel.

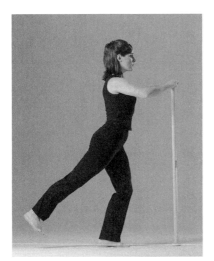

6. Plié, bending both knees,
and reverse the pattern,
reaching your leg to the
back, 4 times.

7. Repeat with the other leg.

H E L P F U L   R E M I N D E R S :

- This movement is flowing and precise, creating a half circle or the letter D.
- Keep your hips down and your back erect as you circle with straight legs and bent knees.
- Slide your working foot against the floor as you come back to your standing parallel position.

Passé and Balance

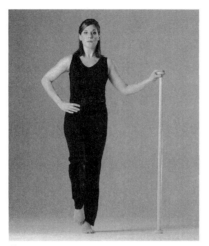 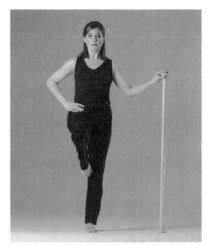

1. Inhale. From your parallel position, draw your right foot up the inside of your left (supporting) leg, starting at the ankle, or at coupé up to passé, just beneath the knee. Place your hand on your hip, keeping your sides long.

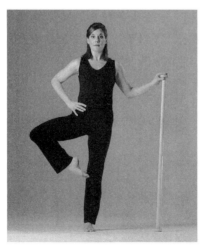 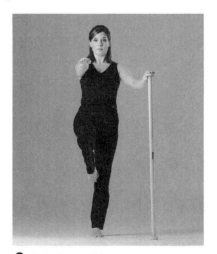

2. Exhale, pull up, and tighten your buttocks. Rotate your knee in passé position to turn out, keeping your hips facing front. In your passé position, turn in and out 4 times.

3. Inhale, and bring your knee back to passé in parallel. Extend your right arm in front at chest level, directly in line with the knee.

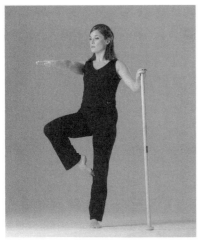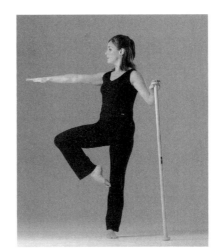

4. Exhale, and follow your arm and knee as you rotate your torso
to the opposite corner, or to 120 degrees. Press your knee away,
and lift your weight out of your hips.

5. Inhale, and slowly follow your arms, keeping your torso and knees
in line back to parallel passé position.

6. Repeat this sequence 4 times on each leg.

HELPFUL REMINDERS:

- Always keep your back long and abdominal muscles lifted as you slide your foot up, down, open, and close.
- Your standing leg, inner thighs, and quadriceps should be activated to take pressure out of your ankles, knees, and hips.
- Keep your chest lifted and shoulders back.
- Ground your feet and stay in parallel.
- Hold the BalleCore Barre or Band horizontal at chest level to challenge your balance further.

Fondue—Lunge—Warrior III

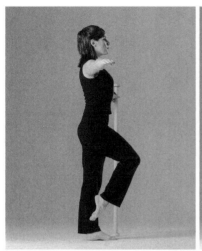 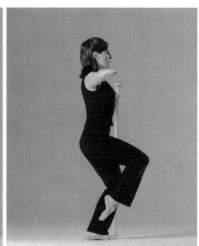 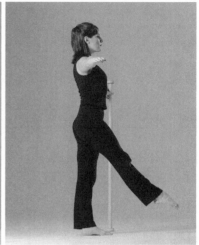

1. Inhale, and, in your parallel position, extend your right arm to the side with your palms facing down. Draw your right foot just above your ankle at coupé, and point your toes.

2. Exhale, bend your supporting (left) leg, or plié, and keep your right foot at the ankle, to fondue. Your back stays lifted.

3. Inhale, stretch, and extend both legs simultaneously. Repeat the fondue 6 times.

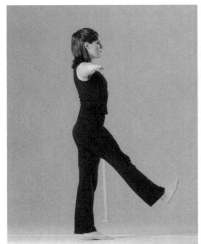 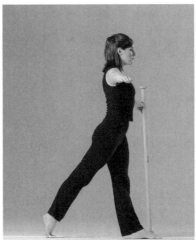 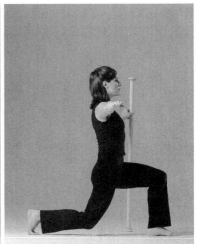

4. Flex your foot and point, several times.

5. Draw your right foot to your left ankle and extend your right leg to the back. Place the ball of your right foot down. Find equal weight on both legs.

6. In your lunge position, lower your back knee, keeping your front knee over your ankle and at a right angle.

(continued on next page)

Fondue—Lunge—Warrior III (continued)

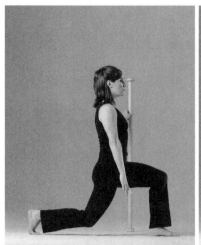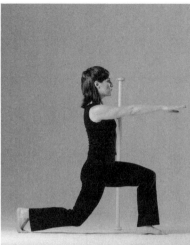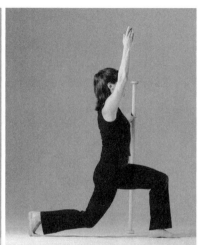

7. Using both legs in your lunge position, slowly pulse your legs only a few inches up and down. Simultaneously port de bras your right arm, making a large circle. Follow this port de bras pattern: side—down—front—overhead—side. Repeat twice.

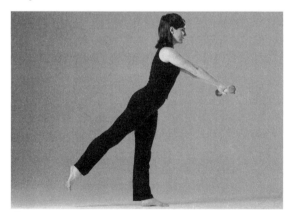

8. Straighten the right leg, pushing through the ball of your foot. Testing your balance, switch the BalleCore Barre to chest level, horizontally. Breathe deeply and focus inward. Using your core support, lift your back leg and slowly shift your upper body forward. Push off the floor with your left leg, as you energize and pull up with your inner thighs.

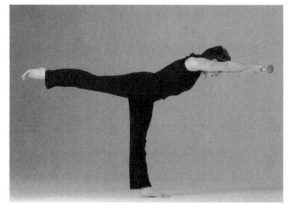

9. Finding balance, continue to lift the back leg out and up as the crown of your head reaches forward. Try to bring your body parallel to the floor in one straight line.

Fondue—Lunge—Warrior III: With Chair

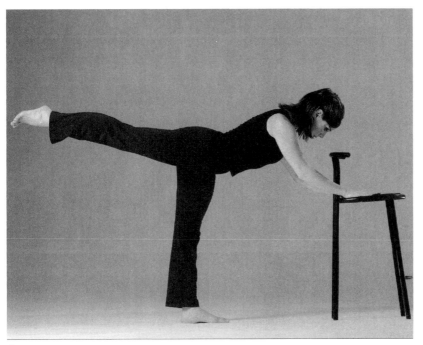

1. Use a chair to practice, or to hold the BalleCore Barre vertically.

HELPFUL REMINDERS:

- To maintain full body control with this variation, stay focused and engage all your muscle groups, emanating from your core.

- *Fondue* means "to melt." Relax your knee joints as you bend. As you straighten both legs, pull the front of your thighs up. This will lift and stabilize your kneecaps.

- Keep these movements connected and seamless.

- Lunging properly requires you to remain centered. Do not shift forward or sit back as you pulse during lunges. Drop your tailbone and lift your abdominals.

- As you coordinate your port de bras arms with lunges, breathe in and out as you fully extend the arms and fingers through all your arm positions.

- During Warrior III Pose, keep your hips and shoulders facing forward. Feel your standing foot rooted into the floor, and your inner thighs and groin engaged. Balance on top of your hips rather than sinking weight into the left hip. Feel long.

Passé—Développé—

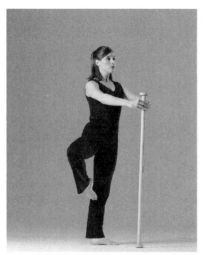 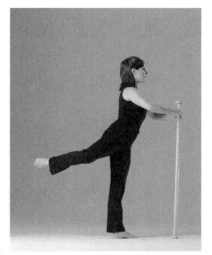

1. Stand in your turn-out position. Inhale. Draw your right foot up the inside of your left (supporting) leg starting at the ankle, or at coupé up to passé, just beneath your knee. Place both hands on your BalleCore Barre or a chair.

2. Exhale, pull up, and tighten your buttocks. Rotate your knee from passé position to the back, keeping your knee bent, without dropping the level of your back knee. This is attitude position to the back.

Ballet Lunge—Arabesque

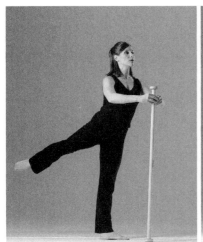 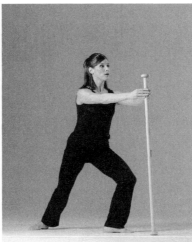 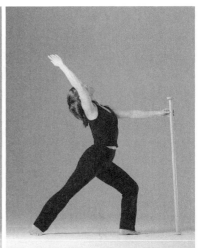

3. Inhale. At 45 degrees, fully extend the back leg, reaching out of your hip to développé. Stretch through your toes. Keep your chest lifted.

4. Bend your front knee, take a large step back, and lower your right foot. This is your fourth position ballet lunge.

5. Bring your right arm up to a fifth port de bras and lift upward out of your hips. Now bend your back or cambré backward and look up.

(continued on next page)

Passé—Développé—

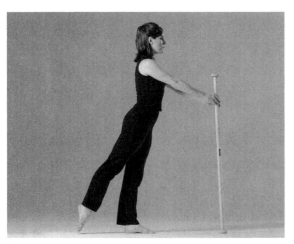

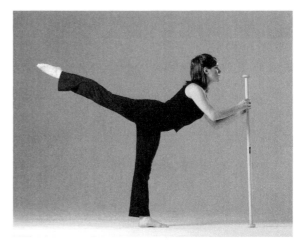

6. Straighten your front leg and stretch your back leg to tendu.

7. Slightly shift your upper body forward as you lift your back leg off the floor, keeping your knee straight. Continue to heighten your back leg to your final extension, at the same time increasing the tilt of the upper body to accommodate your extension. Hold this position for several seconds.

8. Slowly lower your back leg as you lift your torso up and point your foot to tendu.

Ballet Lunge—Arabesque (continued)

HELPFUL REMINDERS:

- As you passé and move into attitude to the back, do not allow your hip to hike up.

- Your back muscles will be firing while you work on leg extension.

- In arabesque, maintain a strong, lifted upper back and keep your shoulders back. You should remain long.

- Your arabesque will heighten over time as you strengthen your back and legs and increase mobility in your spine through stretching. Begin with your leg just a few inches off the floor and work from there.

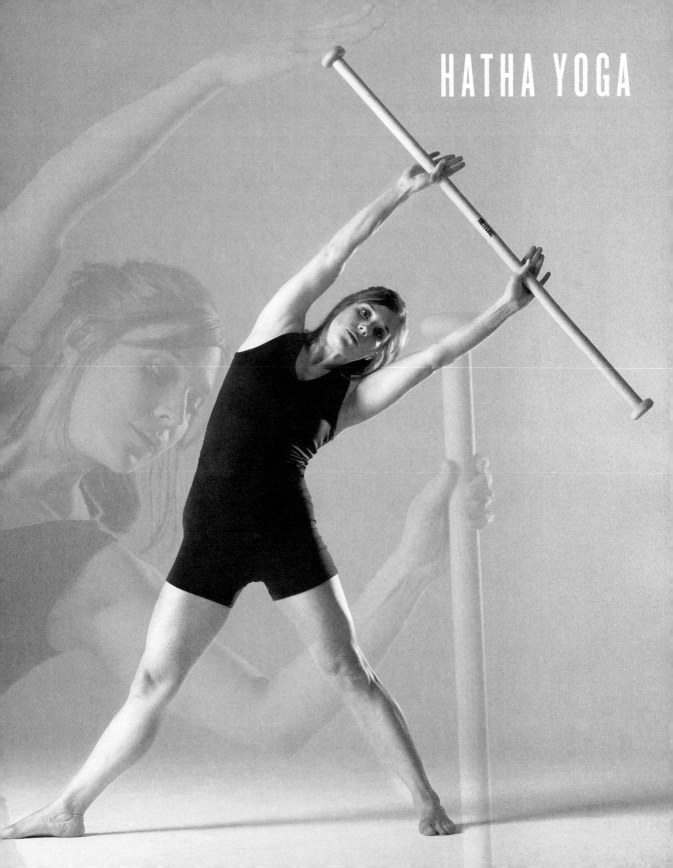

Hatha Yoga

Bringing a sense of lightness through your body is a great way to imagine the next series of exercises. The movements are large-range positions that require you to use your muscular strength rather than relying on the ligaments. These exercises can be quite challenging, but a determined mind-set and an aligned body–mind–spirit can help you achieve surprising results. Fluid breathing should be linked to each position, relieving stiffness in the body and allowing you to build stamina as you hold these postures for several breaths.

Benefits:

- ❑ Builds stamina and confidence.
- ❑ Strengthens entire body.

WARRIOR II AND SIDE ANGLE WITH PORT DE BRAS VARIATION:

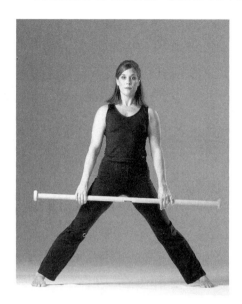

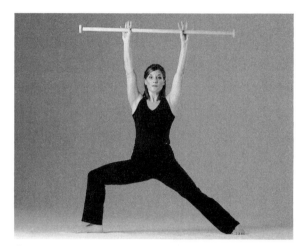

1. Starting in your parallel position, feel tall, centered, and supported by your core. Jump or step out between 4 and 5 feet. Your toes are facing front. Rest your barre against the fronts of your thighs. Keep your hips facing front.

2. Turn your right foot out by pivoting on your heel to 90 degrees. Your toes are spread and your entire leg is stretched outward. Place your right (front) heel in direct line with the back (left) arch of your foot. Your back (left) foot is turned inward. Bend your right knee directly over your right ankle and in line with your big toe.

3. Inhale, lift your barre overhead, and reach out of your waist.

4. Exhale, and bring your barre down to your hips. Inhale, and bring your barre back up overhead.

5. Repeat, lifting the barre up and down 4 times.

With BalleCore Barre

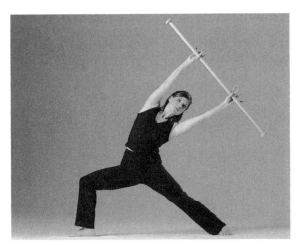

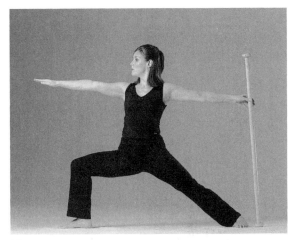

6. Exhale, and bend your torso sideways to the left or cambré with your barre overhead.

7. Release your barre by gently allowing it to slide down your hands. Line your barre up with your left foot. Extend your right arm in direct line with your leg and reach. Hold your Warrior II Pose for several seconds. Breathe in and out.

(continued on next page)

WARRIOR II AND SIDE ANGLE WITH PORT DE BRAS VARIATION:

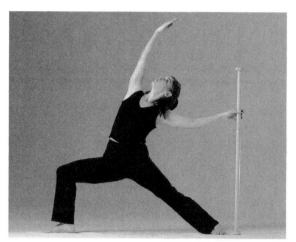 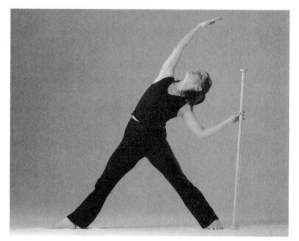

8. Turn your palm to face up, and follow your hand as you bend your right side to Reverse Warrior Pose. Keep your front knee bent at a right angle. Continue to breathe naturally.

9. Straighten your front leg and continue to bend over or cambré to the side. Feel a stretch through your heel, up your leg, and out through your fingertips.

With BalleCore Barre (continued)

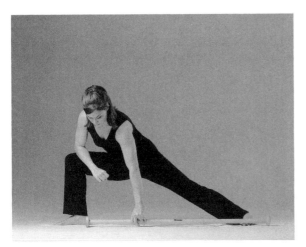

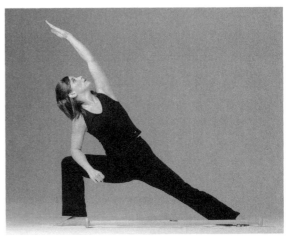

10. Bend your front knee and lower your barre. Bring your knee back over your front ankle and in line with your toes so it is in proper alignment.

11. Rest your right forearm on your upper thigh. Use your arm to rotate your hips farther outward. Stretch and raise your left arm up to your ear. Look at the crease of your elbow. Your body should form one straight diagonal line from your back heel through your fingertips. Breathe in and out and hold Side Angle Pose. Repeat on the other side.

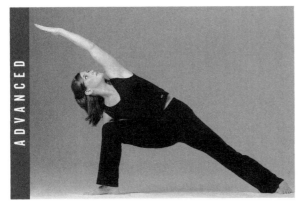

1. Bring your palm to the floor and reach the right arm farther forward, creating a longer diagonal. Gaze at your fingertips and hold the pose.

WARRIOR II AND SIDE ANGLE WITH PORT DE BRAS VARIATION:

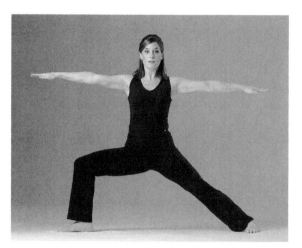 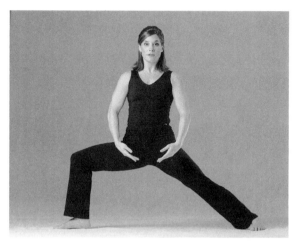

1. Follow steps 1 and 2 on page 224 without the barre.
2. Extend both arms out to your sides. Your wrists should be directly over your ankles. Your palms should face down. Inhale and exhale.

3. Exhale. Bring your arms down, and round the elbows in just in front of your hips.

Without BalleCore Barre

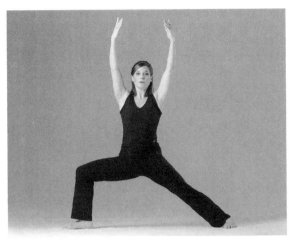 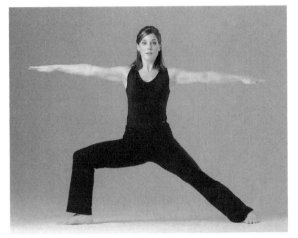

4. Inhale, and move your arms through port de bras, from your center to overhead. Draw your shoulders down.

5. Exhale, and bring your arms out to the sides and down to your hips. Inhale, and bring your arms back overhead.

6. Repeat your port de bras arms moving up to the sides and down, 4 times.

(continued on next page)

WARRIOR II AND SIDE ANGLE WITH PORT DE BRAS VARIATION:

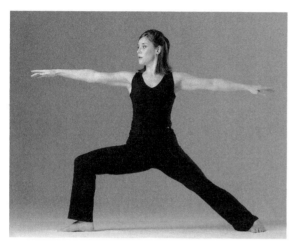 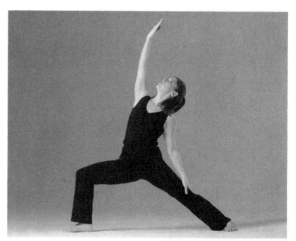

7. Stretch your arms again out to the sides, keeping your hips facing front. Exhale, turn your head to look beyond the right hand. Hold Warrior II for several seconds.

8. Turn your palm to face up, and follow your hand as you bend your right side to Reverse Warrior Pose. Keep your front knee bent. Continue to breathe naturally.

HELPFUL REMINDERS:

- This variation heats and invigorates the body. Stamina increases with practice.
- These poses release the deeper inner muscles of the pelvis, hips, and back as they strengthen the lower body.
- Feel balanced by maintaining equal weight with both feet and legs throughout the sequence.
- As you bend your front knee at a right angle, make sure the knee is in line with your ankle and big toe.
- As you descend, feel light by pulling up out of your waist with the upper half of your body.
- Keep rotating your shoulders back and broaden your back to increase width and length in the upper body while in Side Angle Pose.

Without BalleCore Barre (continued)

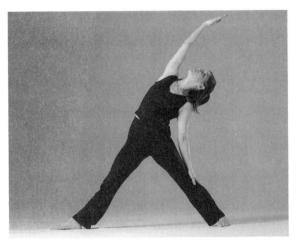

9. Straighten your front leg and continue to bend or cambré to the side. Feel a stretch starting from your heel, up your leg, and out through your fingertips.

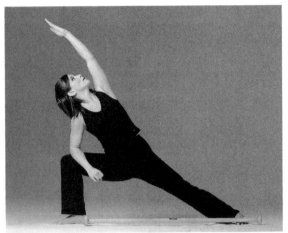

10. Bend your front knee. Bring your knee back over your front ankle and in line with your toes so it is in proper alignment. Rest your right forearm on your upper thigh. Use your arm to rotate your hips farther outward. Stretch and raise your left arm up to your ear. Look at the crease of your elbow. Your body should form one straight diagonal line from your back heel through your fingertips. Breathe in and out and hold Side Angle Pose. Repeat on the other side.

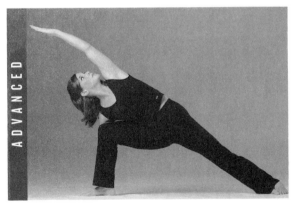

ADVANCED

1. Bring your palm to the floor and reach the right arm farther forward, creating a longer diagonal. Gaze at your fingertips and hold the pose.

Straddle Torso Twist

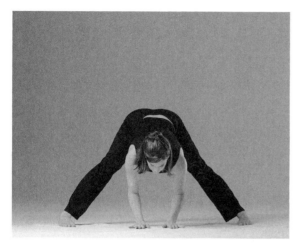
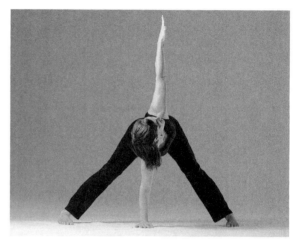

1. Stretch your legs out about 4 to 5 feet wide. Bend forward and exhale. Press your hands firmly into the floor in line with your toes. Keep your elbows wide. Maintain a long line from head to tail while maintaining a flat back.

2. Press your right hand firmly in the floor at the center of your body. Inhale and exhale as you rotate your left arm, upper back, and chest toward the ceiling. Look up at your thumb.

HELPFUL REMINDERS:

- In your straddle position, keep your feet and knees facing front as you draw your thigh muscles up, taking pressure out of your knees. Lift your tailbone and sitting bones upward.
- Narrow the width of your stance if the stretch in your hamstrings is too uncomfortable.
- Slightly turn your toes inward to prevent slipping.
- Firmly place your palms into the floor and energize the arms as you rotate into a long straight line.
- When you rotate your trunk, feel the expansion across the chest, as your shoulder reaches away from you.

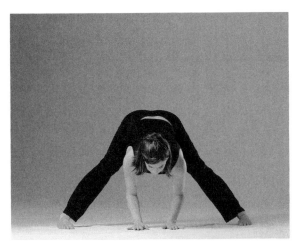

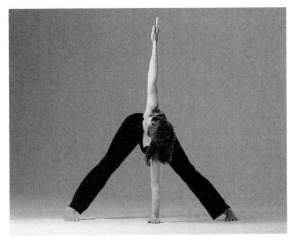

3. Inhale, and bring your palms back to the floor. Press your hands firmly into the floor at the center of your body.

4. Exhale, and rotate your left arm as it reaches up toward the ceiling. Look up to your thumb.

5. Reach for your barre and straighten your body.

6. Jump or step back to parallel position.

REPEAT 2 TIMES

NAMASTE FORWARD BEND VARIATION:

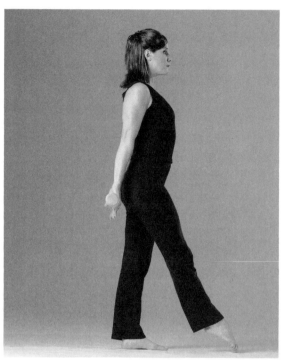 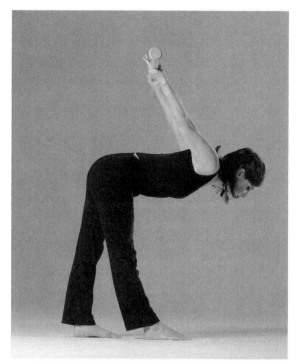

1. Standing in parallel, bring the BalleCore Barre behind you with your palms facing out toward the floor. Point your right foot and lower your heel. Feel equal weight on both legs.

2. Inhale, reach your barre away, and lift it up, keeping your chest open as you start your forward bend. Exhale, continue to bend forward, and reach the barre up to the ceiling. Maintain a flat back and shift your front hip bone back in line to meet your other hip bone.

With BalleCore Barre

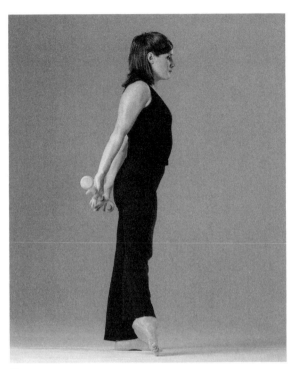 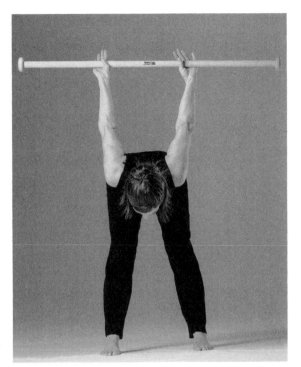

3. Inhale, come out of your forward bend, and lift up. Tendu front. Rond de jambe your foot in parallel, to the side. Place your foot down.

4. Exhale, and bend forward, reaching the barre up to the ceiling. Maintain a flat back and take weight out of your hip bones by pulling up and utilizing your core.

5. Inhale, come out of your forward bend, and lift up.

6. Repeat with your other leg.

NAMASTE FORWARD BEND VARIATION: *Bound Arms*

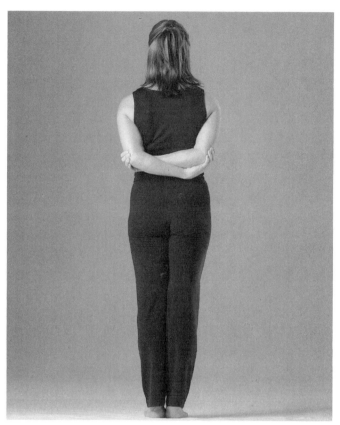

1. Bend your right arm and take it behind your back. Hold your left arm at your elbow or forearm, and take it back to bind the arms. Keep your back erect and your shoulders back.

NAMASTE FORWARD BEND VARIATION: *Namaste Arms*

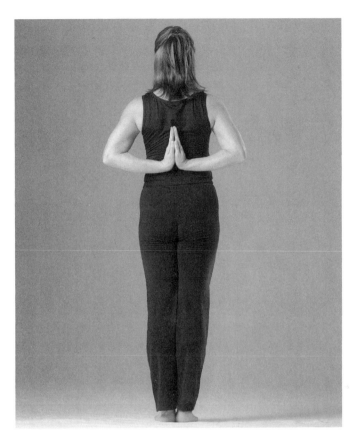

1. Take your arms behind you and join your fingers and palms together. Move your elbows back and slide your palms to face up and together.

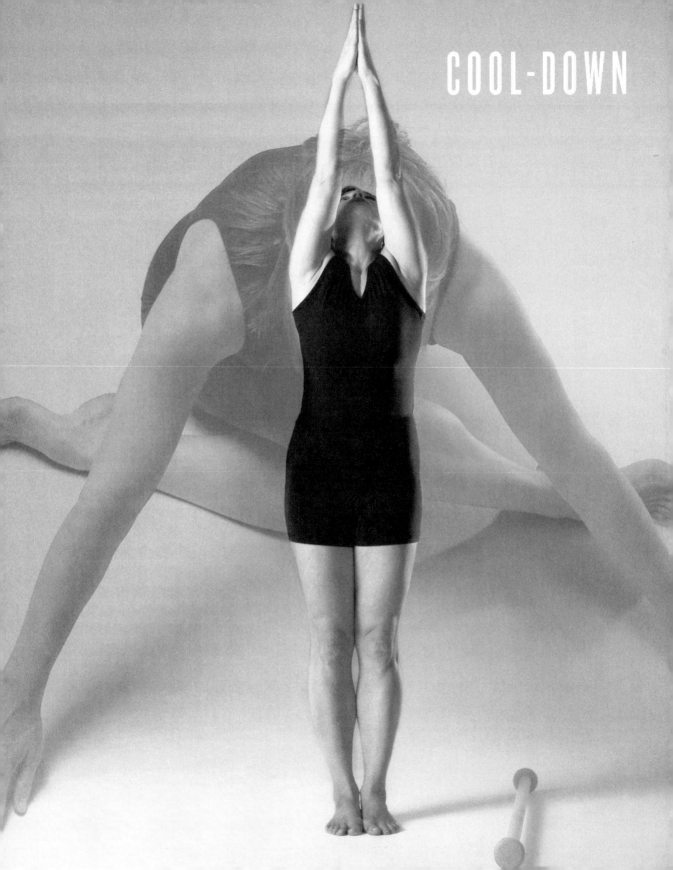

Cool-Down

To help you restore mental, emotional, and physical balance, cool-down exercises are important to lead the body and mind to a state of calmness. Let go of unwanted tension, quieting the body from the inside out as you slow down with these exercises. This part of the workout will replenish your physical energy and motivate you to return.

Benefits:

❑ Releases tension in the body.
❑ Renews energy.
❑ Centers the muscles and mind.

Point-and-Flex Stretch

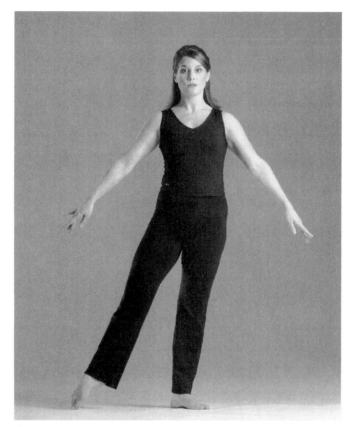

1. In your first position, extend your arms out into a low V position. Extend your right leg and stretch your foot out to tendu to the side.

HELPFUL REMINDERS:

- Slightly shift your weight into your supporting leg as you stretch and flex your working foot.
- Stretching your feet after vigorous standing postures helps avoid cramps in the calves and ankles.
- As you tendu to the side, your leg and foot are extended in line with your hip bone.

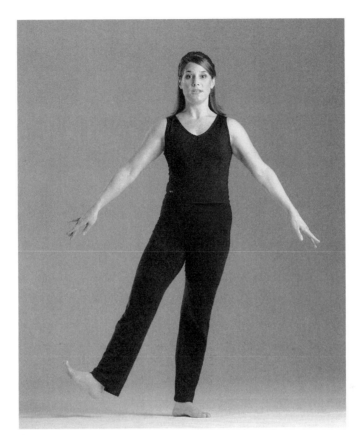

2. Flex the foot and point the foot off the floor. Keep your balance. Repeat pointing and flexing 6 times.

3. Bring your foot back to your first position.

4. Repeat on the other side.

Standing Shoulder Release

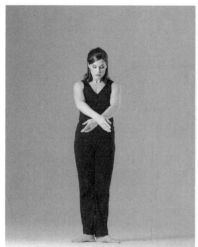 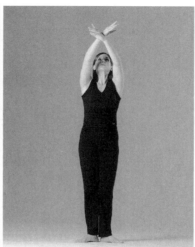 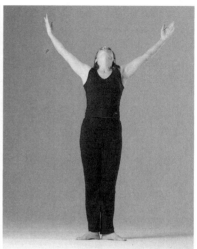

1. In your first position, lower your head and cross your arms to start. Inhale and bring your arms up the center of your body, crossing at your wrists.

2. Continue to carry your arms up overhead. Stretch your neck and look up to your wrists.

3. Open your chest and slightly bend back. Let your arms open to a wide V position.

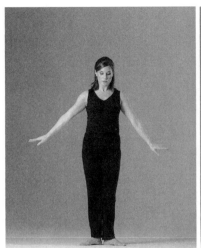 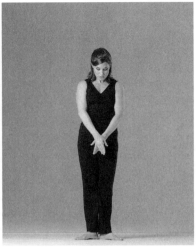

4. Exhale, turn your palms to face down, and bring your arms back to cross in front at your waist. Reverse your arms and follow steps 1 to 4.

REPEAT 2 TIMES

HELPFUL REMINDERS:

- Your elbows and wrists should be slightly rounded as you move your arms and open your shoulders.
- Feel your upper back and chest expanding and continuing to release each time.
- Slowly, yet with energy, move your arms.
- Focus on breathing with ease.

Upward Stretch

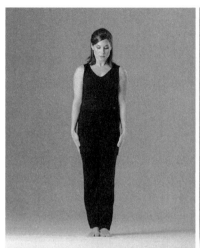 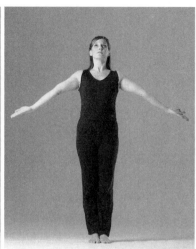 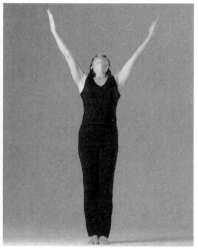

1. Start in parallel position with your arms at your sides and eyes down. Feel centered.

2. Inhale, and reach your arms out to the sides with your palms facing up. Look up.

3. Continue to inhale and reach your arms up overhead.

HELPFUL REMINDERS:

- Energize your arms as you stretch.
- Keep your inner thighs tight as you stretch up and down with the arms.
- Feel your body strong, centered, and light as you cool down inside and out.

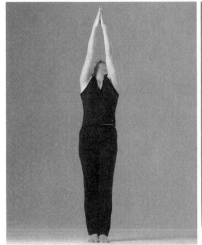

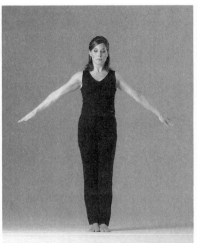

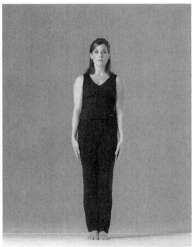

4. Bring your palms together and hold the stretch.

5. Exhale and press your arms away to lower them.

6. Look straight ahead with your arms at your sides, and bring your breathing back to normal.

REPEAT 3 TIMES

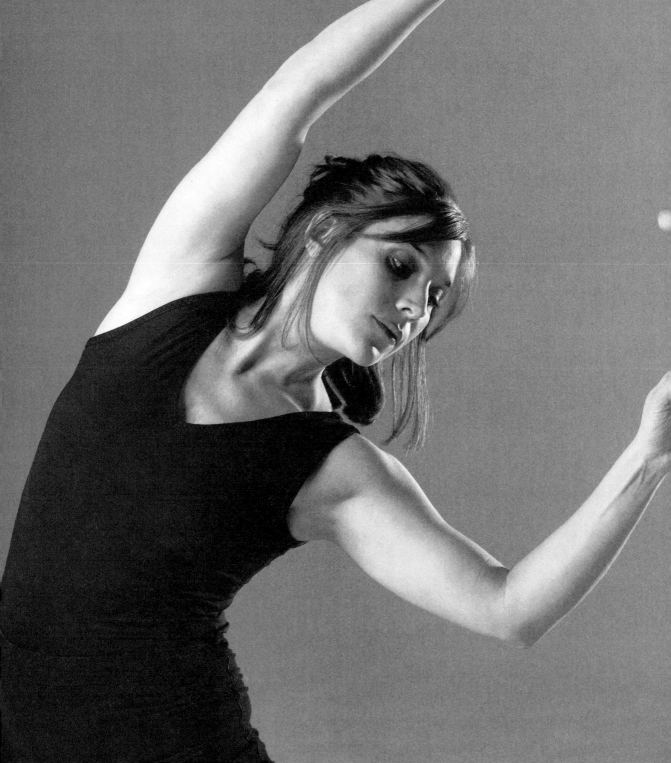

BALLECORE TIME-SAVERS

BalleCore Time-Savers

Is your schedule hectic, due to family obligations or last-minute projects at the office? If you don't want to miss out on exercising but simply cannot schedule enough time for yourself, a BalleCore Time-Saver is your answer! I have designed shortened routines so that you can take care of yourself in half the time or less. They require only 10 minutes of time, mental focus, and determination. These specially designed programs can help you maintain a healthy body and mind when your day won't allow you the time for the complete 50-minute workout. The four programs I outline below are modified versions of the complete BalleCore program. For instance, if you are on vacation and want to relax, I recommend the BalleCore Express, which only takes 20 minutes. The Express is also the perfect place for the careful beginner to start. Once you're comfortable with the Express exercises, feel free to add and tailor the program to make it more challenging, or to focus on a particular area. It's okay to build and progress toward the full, seamless 50-minute routine in whatever way you choose, but to be true to the flow of BalleCore, always keep the exercises in the order you find them in the main program—the sequencing is important to experience the overall benefits.

You can also easily choose one of the other 10- or 15-minute BalleCore programs. Though each has a specific focus, you should know that more than one muscle group is involved with each exercise and there is an array of benefits to each. These shortened routines are also a perfect complement to playing sports. For instance, all golfers work at improving their swing. To generate more speed and rotation in the trunk, the 15-Minute Hip Opener is the key to improving your game. The Hip Opener program is designed to increase mobility in your hips and flexibility in your back. Alternating Time-Savers is also another way to keep fit during hectic times. I recommend this routine: On Monday, try the 10-Minute Core Strengthener; on Tuesday, sample the BalleCore Express; on Wednesday, tackle the 15-Minute Hip Opener; on Thursday, go back to the BalleCore Express; and on Friday, test your balance with the 10-Minute Balance Challenge. Whatever your reason may be for not having 50 minutes to exercise, any of these quick programs will keep you motivated and feeling spectacular!

THE 20-MINUTE BALLECORE EXPRESS

If you are a beginner or on the go and don't have the time for the full 50-minute routine, the BalleCore Express program is a great way to achieve the same results in less than half the time. Key moves from the complete BalleCore Workout have been chosen to work your body inside and out. There are 25 exercises in all.

Floor Exercises

Standing Exercises

THE 10-MINUTE CORE STRENGTHENER

In just 10 minutes you can simultaneously save your back and firm your abs. These eight very effective exercises target the body's core. Attention to form and proper breathing can help prevent back pain and develop dynamic power in your body's center.

THE 10-MINUTE BALANCE CHALLENGE

Investing in 10 minutes of balance training will pay off whether you are a novice or athlete. Balance is the foundation for all movement, and after the age of 25, our sense of equilibrium diminishes. I recommend practicing these eight exercises to ultimately improve coordination, posture, and full body control.

THE 15-MINUTE HIP OPENER

If your hips are tight, did you know that problems can result in other areas, such as lower back pain or tight hamstrings? Zero in on the hips with these eight moves to stretch and open up the front, sides, and back of the hip ultimately creating a more balanced body.

STRETCHING

HIPS AND BUTTOCKS

  Repeat with your other leg.

HATHA YOGA

  If you do not have a BalleCore Barre, do this variation 4 times with port de bras arms.

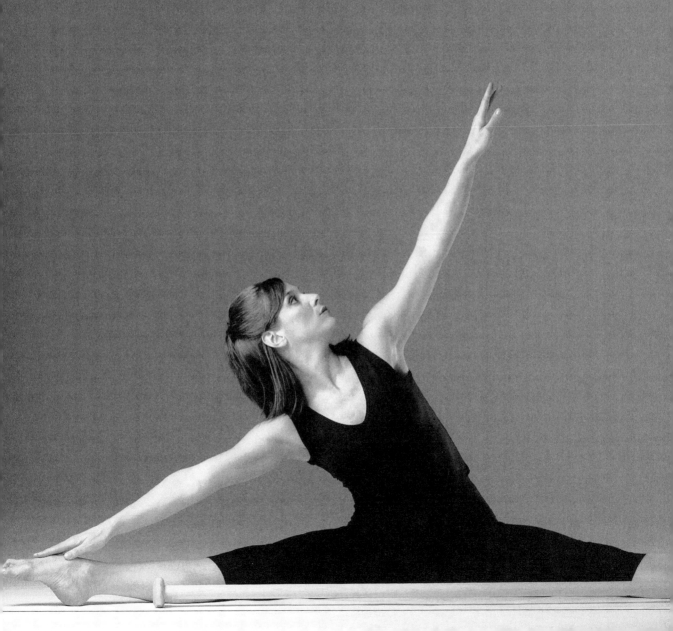

GLOSSARY

General Terms

Connection to the mat: The muscles that run along the spine (paraspinal) muscles and muscles of respiration are relaxed. Awareness is brought to the center, and the central nervous system is calm, preparing the body and mind for the floor exercises.

Extension: Stretching out. Bending backward (as in the Cobra).

Flexion: Bending, curling the body forward (as in Roll-Up exercises).

Head-lifted, curl-up position: The core muscles are engaged and proper breathing is incorporated as the neck is in flexion. Head, neck, and shoulder blades are lifted off the floor, keeping the base of the scapulae in contact with the floor. In this correct position, the torso can be flexed, contracting the abdominals to slide the rib cage toward the pelvis. The pelvis is slightly imprinted.

Imprint position: A slightly tilted pelvis, which brings the lower back into the floor.

Navel to spine: The physical and mental act of connecting the abdominals to the spine to protect the core and center the body.

Neutral position: The hip bones and pubic bone are on the same plane. Cue for correct placement.

Opposition: When the arm position is opposite that of the working leg.

Pilates V: A Pilates posture in which feet are in a narrow V position, with heels together and toes apart. The inner thighs and gluteal muscles are engaged to assist with full body control.

Posture and alignment check: The weight of the body is correctly centered over the feet, with weight equal between the heels and balls of the feet, kneecaps lifted, inner thighs engaged, pelvis neutral, abdominal muscles pulled in and up, scapulaes drawn down, and neck long and balanced on top of shoulders.

Pulled up: The weight of the body is lifted away from the floor during the standing ballet work. This is done by engaging the leg and core muscles. (Pulling up during the standing ballet work is essential.)

Rotation: Turning around; to move around the axis of a bone.

Scapular placement: To maintain stability in the shoulder area. The scapulae are drawn down the back and toward the spine in a V position. The width between the shoulders and chest is broadened.

Turn-out position: Rotation of the feet and legs, turned out from the hip joint.

Ballet Terms

Arabesque: Body held upright, supported on one leg, with the other leg extended behind at a right angle.

Attitude: Knee bent at a 90-degree angle and higher than the foot.

Battement: The working leg is raised from the hip into the air and brought down again.

Cambré: A bend of the body from the waist, forward, sideways, or backward.

Coupé: "Cut." The foot is lifted to the other ankle.

Dégagé: "Disengaged." A strong pointed foot brushes in an open position, lifting off the floor.

Demi-pointe: The foot points three-quarters of the way. The action of gently pushing through the base of the toes and ball of the foot. (This is used in many BalleCore exercises to lengthen the leg muscle.)

Développé: The working leg slides up the opposite knee and fully extends.

Flexed foot: Pushing through the heel and toes to the ceiling.

Fondue: "To melt, or sinking down." Bend to spring and align on one leg.

Grand plié (in second position): A larger knee bend. The heels remain on the floor.

Passé: Sliding the foot up the inside of the supporting leg to the knee.

Penché: Tilting of the body. Ideal position for a 180° split.

Piqué: Toes tapping the floor, and the leg lifts to 45 degrees.

Plié: Bending of the knees.

Pointed foot: The ankle is held strong in a vertical position. The foot is fully extended.

Port de bras: "The carriage of arms." A series of movements made by passing the arms through various positions. The arms, not the shoulders, move gracefully and expressively, in harmony with the rest of the body.

Relevé: "Raised." Lift the heels up to the balls of the feet; also referred to as *demi-pointe*.

Rond de jambe: A circular movement of the leg, making the letter D.

Sous-sus: "Under-over." One foot is crossed over the other in fifth position and on relevé (used in side-lying exercises in BalleCore).

Tendu: Stretched, arched foot.

FOR MORE INFORMATION

To purchase a BalleCore Barre or BalleCore Band, visit www.ballecore.com and order online.

To find out more about BalleCore classes in the United States, Europe, Puerto Rico, Canada, Brazil, and Australia, visit www.ballecore.com for listings of classes and instructors in your area. BalleCore is currently taught at dance and Pilates studios, universities, community centers, destination spas, and fitness clubs.

If you are interested in becoming a BalleCore instructor and wish to find out more about the certification process and licensing, all the information you need is available at www.ballecore.com

INDEX

ABOUT THE AUTHOR

Molly Weeks, creator of BalleCore®, is a nationally recognized fitness professional and has been a faculty member of the Boston Ballet for the past seven years. She has taught extensively throughout the United States, including fitness industry events, universities, adult education centers, health clubs, dance centers, and destination spas. BalleCore has been featured in *Self* magazine, *Newsweek*, *Harper's Bazaar*, *The Boston Globe* and *The Washington Post*. BalleCore is one of the fastest growing exercise programs worldwide. Molly trains instructors to teach the BalleCore Workout and was a featured presenter at the Pilates Method Alliance international conference in 2004. She lives in the Boston area with her husband and two daughters.